Living Fit

Living Fit

Henry J. Montoye
Janet L. Christian
Francis J. Nagle
Saul M. Levin

University of Wisconsin–Madison

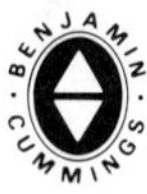

The Benjamin/Cummings Publishing Company, Inc.
Menlo Park, California • Reading, Massachusetts • Don Mills, Ontario •
Wokingham, U.K. • Amsterdam • Sydney • Singapore •
Tokyo • Madrid • Bogota • Santiago • San Juan

Sponsoring Editor: Connie Spatz
Production Editor: Katherine Brock/Science Tech Publishers
Production Coordinator: Janet Vail
Text Design: Katherine Brock
Cover Design: Gary Head
Art Direction: Katherine Brock/Science Tech Publishers
Illustrations: Tony Dunn, Patricia Jeffson, Lisa Buckley
Copy Editor: Ruth Siegel
Composition: Science Tech Publishers and Impressions, Inc.

Library of Congress Cataloging-in-Publication Data

Living fit.

Includes index.
1. Health behavior. 2. Exercise. 3. Nutrition.
4. Physical fitness. I. Montoye, Henry Joseph.
RA776.9.L58 1988   613   87-32583
ISBN   0-8053-8180-5

BCDEFGHIJ-HA-898

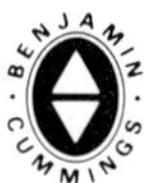

The Benjamin/Cummings Publishing Company, Inc.
2727 Sand Hill Road
Menlo Park, California 94025

To the many college students who want to develop or maintain lifestyles conducive to better physical and mental health,

and to the dedicated teachers who are helping their students achieve this goal.

Preface

This book is about living fit—how to do it, why to do it, and how to get back to living fit after you've stopped for a while.

Living Fit is designed primarily as a textbook for introductory college courses in conditioning, lifestyle modification, fitness, and health. It has evolved during the past seven years as we've developed and co-taught a course called Exercise, Nutrition, and Health at the University of Wisconsin–Madison. We wrote the book because there wasn't one available that adequately addressed the topics we thought most important—how to exercise for health, fun, and safety; how to eat healthfully; how to reduce stress and how to motivate yourself to start a health program and stay with it.

We put the book together in the order in which we currently teach the course. However, it lends itself well to other organizations. We have sometimes addressed the topics in a different order, such as presenting the nutrition material before the exercise component. At other times, we have presented all the background information at the beginning of the course, then provided all of the self-assessment material, then finally the programs. The text is flexible enough to allow for such reorganizations.

Although our own course is in lecture format, the book is equally suited to classes that have a strong physical activity component. If there is not enough time to assign all of the chapters, some can be omitted without destroying the usefulness of the rest. For example, it would be possible to assign the self-assessment and programs chapters on exercise and nutrition (Chapters 4, 5, 9, and 10), while using the background chapters for those areas (Chapters 3 and 8) as reference materials.

Look it over; we think you'll find this book as useful, flexible, and adaptable as a healthy body.

Special features of this book

Here are some features that make this book worth your consideration.

- *This book was written by specialists in the fields of exercise physiology, nutrition, and psychology.* In many cases, fitness books are written by one or more authors whose home turf is limited to physiology. In contrast, our team includes authors with nutrition and psychology expertise, as well as exercise physiology specialists.

  The authors include Henry J. Montoye and Francis J. Nagle, exercise physiologists and professors in the Department of Physical Education and Dance; Janet L. Christian, a registered dietitian and nutrition lecturer whose primary appointment is in the Department of Nutritional Sciences; and Saul M. Levin, a psychologist who not only teaches but also works with patients in state hospital and private practice settings.

  Although this is an authoritative book, it is not difficult. It was written for the reader who has not formally studied these topics before, and it can be used with confidence by instructors whose backgrounds do not encompass all of these disciplines.

- *This book offers suggestions about how to succeed in changing exercise and eating habits.* Many people attempt to change their lifestyles at one time or another but their efforts often fizzle out fast. They may have reasonable goals but be using the wrong methods to achieve them. Here, we will suggest methods from the field of psychology that substantially increase a person's chances of success.

- *This book speaks to the individual.* We recognize that everybody is unique. Some individuals who read this book may have avoided thinking about their fitness for a long time; others may have already taken steps to improve their exercise and eating habits. *Living Fit* speaks to people at both ends of the spectrum and to everybody in between.

  In "self-check" sections throughout the book, we offer frequent opportunities for readers to find out how fit they are. Further, the chapters that deal with programs for improvement do not prescribe a standard program for everyone. Rather, they describe how people can construct individualized programs from easy-to-follow guidelines.

- *Words and drawings tell the story.* For many topics, it is best to communicate with words; for others, illustrations are very effective. In this book, we have emphasized the approach which does the best job, section by section.

Acknowledgments

People who work in physical education and health care are well aware of the value of team effort. Writing a book is another experience that makes one appreciate the importance of teamwork.

Not only are we referring to the team of authors involved in this project, but also to the talented people at Benjamin/Cummings who lent their skills to this project. We want to thank Diane Bowen and Robin Williams, who initially took turns shouldering editorial responsibilities for this book. We also gratefully acknowledge the yeoman's task done by associate editor Langdon Faust, who held our project to the refiner's fire and attended to innumerable editorial details. Kathie and Tom Brock and their staff at Science Tech Publishers deserve kudos for producing the book in a timely fashion.

We also wish to thank Frederick F. Andres of the University of Toledo in Ohio, Elizabeth Anne Frechette of the University of South Carolina in Columbia, Edward T. Howley of the University of Tennessee in Knoxville, and Jane Roberts of Mankato State University in Minnesota for their careful reviews. Their helpful suggestions at various points along the way enhanced the quality of this book.

Henry J. Montoye
Janet L. Christian
Francis J. Nagle
Saul M. Levin

ABOUT THE AUTHORS OF LIVING FIT

Henry J. Montoye, PhD, is a distinguished scholar and life-long participant in a variety of sports. He has held academic positions at Michigan State University, the University of Michigan, the University of Tennessee, and the University of Wisconsin–Madison, where he has twice served as department chair. He is active in many professional organizations and served as president of the American Academy of Physical Eduction and the American College of Sports Medicine. Among many honors awarded him, he was the first Alliance Scholar named by the American Association for Health, Physical Education, and Recreation.

Janet L. Christian is a Registered Dietitian who began her career in hospital clinical dietetics. Currently a lecturer in the University of Wisconsin–Madison's Department of Nutritional Sciences, she has taught nutrition to over 9,000 nonmajors; in 1986, she was awarded a citation for excellence in teaching. In addition to this book, she has coauthored with Professor Janet Greger a leading nonmajors nutrition text entitled *Nutrition for Living*.

Francis J. Nagle, PhD, brings a rich background of education and experience to his current position as Professor of Physiology and Physical Education at the University of Wisconsin–Madison. He has earned academic degrees in administration, physical education, and physiology. His varied positions have included being a professional football player, a college football and baseball coach, Chief of the Biodynamics Evaluation Section for the Federal Aviation Agency, and Director of the UW Biodynamics Laboratory.

Saul M. Levin, PhD psychologist, has a full three-part career as a private practitioner in psychology, Head of the Psychophysiology Laboratory at Mendota Mental Health Institute, and lecturer at the University of Wisconsin–Madison. Major professional interests include helping people acquire behaviors that maintain health and reduce risk factors for disease and using behavioral approaches to treat anxiety and depression.

Table of Contents

Your Health in Today's World — 1

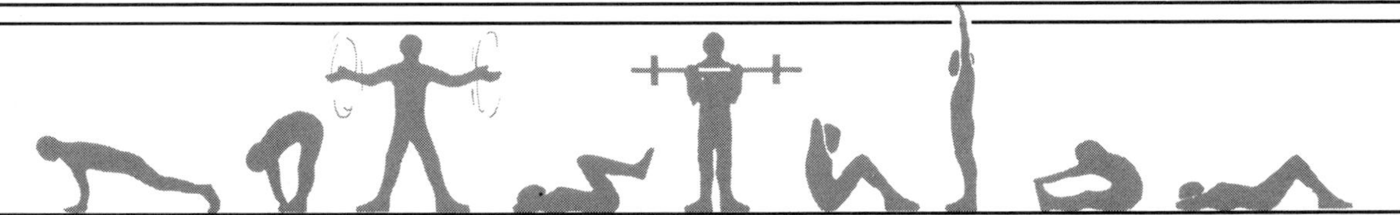

Outline

We assume that you are a typical young or middle-aged adult. You have known what it's like to feel good.

Think back to some occasion when life felt just right. Your alert mind told your body what to do. You felt confident and in control both physically and mentally. The challenges in your life did not bog you down; in fact, you looked forward to dealing with new situations. You were enthusiastic and energetic, eager to live life fully—in a phrase, totally HEALTHY.

How magnificent!

Our culture is full of ideas about how to achieve such vibrant living. The media assault us with all kinds of suggestions: lifting weights; drinking diet soda; cross-country skiing; taking vitamin supplements; meditating; taking stress-reducing, pain-relieving, or other drugs; practicing yoga; losing weight; gaining weight; avoiding processed foods; eating certain foods—these and more are heralded as the means of realizing the sought-after state of health.

Obviously, such diverse suggestions cannot all be on target. A few of those ideas could actually be *un*healthy. Some may focus on short-term "quick fix" or cosmetic changes, rather than on enhancing current and future health; others may be good for certain people but not for everybody. Some may be nothing more than profit-motivated gimmicks.

How can you make sense out of such a scattershot of suggestions, and figure out which ideas (or products or services) might be useful for you?

Providing such help is one of the objectives of this book. But we will deal first and foremost with living habits that promote good health, and identify others that may have negative effects. With the information in these chapters, you should be able to sort out claims you see and hear elsewhere regarding "how to be healthier," and decide for yourself whether a particular idea has merit for you. As part of that effort, this book provides self-checks which you can use to find out how you measure up right now; it then offers programs for improvement or maintenance of fitness and health.

Our work is based on the sciences of physiology, nutrition, and psychology. The living habits we promote in this book are those that researchers in each of these fields believe are beneficial to health. Such judgments are difficult to make, but current methods of investigation enable us to say with greater certainty than ever before which lifestyles provide the greater health payoffs. These findings are the basis for the health education that many health care providers now offer.

Even though we now know a great deal about how to promote good health, we all have genetic limits to what we can accomplish. That is, we are constitutionally restricted in various ways. A few people may be capable of running a 4-minute mile if they train hard to achieve it, but most of us never could run a mile that fast, no matter how much work and determination we might bring to bear. Therefore, each person must establish individualized goals and expectations. Almost everybody can improve his or her health status—but not necessarily at the same rate or up to the same level.

What Is Good Health?

Before we can discuss how to achieve good health, we need to define what health is. In the past, people regarded health as simply being the absence of illness. That idea could be represented like this:

Today we know that there is more to good health than merely *having no obvious illness*. For one thing, we know there are certain measurable physiological and psychological indicators (called **risk factors**) that often precede and predict the development of obvious illness; people

Risk factor: A circumstance statistically associated with a particular disease.

who have risk factors, even though they may not feel ill, cannot be regarded as healthy either.

For example, high blood pressure is a risk factor for heart disease. A person who has high blood pressure may not feel ill, but may be moving toward an obvious health problem such as a heart attack or stroke. With this in mind, it seems important to include the absence (or control) of risk factors as a component of good health.

Another way of looking at health is to look at what level of body function or fitness a person has achieved. By **fitness**, we mean the ability to meet the demands of everyday living—both physiologically and psychologically. For example, a fit person should be able to climb several flights of stairs without becoming winded, or to take an exam without experiencing great stress. Reducing risk factors and achieving fitness often—but not always—go hand in hand.

Taking these additional factors into account, the revised model of **health** can be represented as a continuum that looks like this:

Fitness: The ability to meet the physical and psychological demands of everyday living.

Health: The state of physical and mental fitness in which there are minimal disease risk factors and no obvious illness.

	No obvious illness but	No obvious illness;	No obvious illness; minimal
Obvious	definite	mininal	risk factors;
illness	risk factors	risk factors	fitness

← **Poorest health**   **Best health** →

You may have heard the term "high level wellness" used to refer to the best possible health. However, we prefer to discuss reducing risk and/or improving fitness because we can actually measure these factors.

Changing Health Problems

One reason our concept of health has changed is that the nature of our illnesses has changed. When we read about advances in medicine, we sometimes assume that current technology should make good health possible for everyone. However, no matter how far we progress in solving various kinds of medical problems, each era (and each area of the world) has its own health challenges. As soon as one set of problems comes under control, a new set rises to the top of the list. Let's look at the recent health history of the United States.

At the turn of the century, the most common diseases were the result of infectious organisms which multiplied in unclean environments and caused illnesses such as pneumonia, influenza, tuberculosis, and poliomyelitis. As the first half of the twentieth century progressed, these diseases became considerably less prevalent in this country (although they remained major problems in many parts of the world).

The popular notion is that this improvement in the health of Americans was the result of medical advances including immunization, antibiotics, and "high-tech" diagnostic and therapeutic devices. These advances did, indeed, play a role in the control of some illnesses: few would deny the importance of the Salk vaccine in the control of polio. However, medical advances apparently had little to do with the decline in the incidence of most infectious diseases; the more significant factors were probably improvements in sanitation and nutrition. At any rate, for a combination of reasons, infectious diseases became less of a threat to health and life in the United States than they had been in the early 1900s. But this did not mean that we had fewer health problems—just different ones.

Chronic: Persisting over a long period of time.

Now the health problems that affect the greatest numbers of people here and in other developed countries are mainly long-term, or **chronic**, diseases. Cardiovascular disease (disease of the heart and blood vessels) is the most striking example, but we must also include cancer, diabetes, respiratory diseases, and arthritis. Emotional problems affect large numbers of people as well. Finally, if we add traffic deaths and injuries, particularly among youth, and sexually transmitted diseases such as AIDS, we have accounted for most of our serious widespread health problems.

Lifestyle Affects Health

An unmistakable feature of these contemporary health problems is that most of them are associated with certain living habits. In a classic series of studies begun by Nedra Belloc and Lester Breslow (1972, 1973, 1980), a large number of adults were questioned regarding their personal health practices. These are the habits that were found to be associated with good health:

- Sleeping seven to eight hours a day
- Eating breakfast regularly
- Never or rarely eating between meals
- Currently being at or near ideal weight for height
- Never smoking cigarettes
- Moderate or no use of alcohol
- Regular physical activity

Belloc and Breslow found that people who followed all or most of these practices were in better health than those who engaged in few or none of the listed habits. More importantly, the studies found that a healthy lifestyle predicted future health and length of life. About ten years after the original data were collected, there was a great difference in survival rates of the subjects: men who followed all seven practices had a death rate that was only 28% of those who followed zero to three of these practices. Similar results were obtained for women.

Technically speaking, this study did not prove that the above mentioned habits *cause* good health; it only showed that these habits and good health were *statistically associated with* each other. Nevertheless, one possible reason for this association is that certain lifestyle practices do, in fact, result in good health and longer life. This remains the best explanation, since many subsequent studies have supported this conclusion.

Based on such accumulated evidence, in 1980 the Centers for Disease Control of the U.S. Public Health Service estimated that lifestyle factors are the major cause of lost years of life before age 65 (Figure 1.1). To help people determine whether they have healthy living habits, the U.S. Department of Health and Human Services has developed a test with which people can rate themselves; it appears in Self-check 1.1. Your results on this test can give you an overall idea of where you stand, before we get to more specific assessments in later chapters.

Although all categories of the self-check deal with factors important to longevity, this book will focus only on certain of them; others are not included. For example, you can participate in a community activity

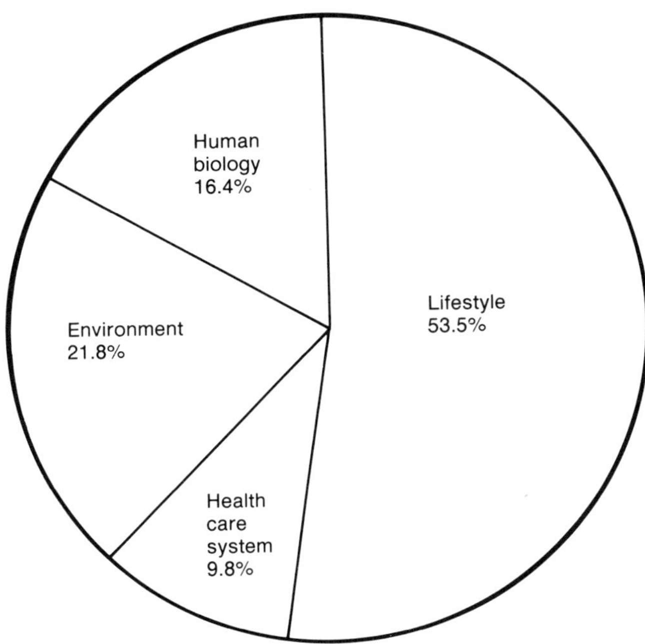

Figure 1.1   Major causes of premature death. This figure shows what proportion of years of life lost in the United States before age 65 are due to various factors. *Human biology* refers mainly to our genetic inheritance: that is, our characteristics and capacities which we cannot change. *Environment* means such factors as air pollution, environmental temperature and humidity, exposure to irradiation, sanitary conditions, etc. *Heath care system* refers to the limitations of our medical system including deaths from incurable diseases, misdiagnoses, insufficient care, etc. Data are based on the ten leading causes of death for people over one year of age.

Self-check 1.1   A test for better health

This is not a pass-fail test. Its purpose is simply to tell you how well you are doing at staying healthy. The behaviors covered in the test are recommended for most Americans. However, some of them may not apply to persons with certain chronic diseases or handicaps. Such persons may require special instructions from their physician or other health professional.

The test has six sections: smoking, alcohol and drugs, nutrition, exercise and fitness, stress control, and safety. Complete one section at a time by circling the number corresponding to the answer that best describes your behavior. Then add the numbers you have circled to determine your score for that section. Write the score on the line provided at the end of each section. The highest score you can get for each section is 10.

	Almost always	Sometimes	Almost never
Cigarette smoking			
If you never smoke, enter a score of 10 for this section and go to the next section on alcohol and drugs			
1. I avoid smoking cigarettes	2	1	0
2. I smoke only low tar and nicotine cigarettes or I smoke a pipe or cigars	2	1	0
Smoking score __________			
Alcohol and drugs			
1. I avoid drinking alcoholic beverages or I drink no more than 1 or 2 drinks a day	4	1	0
2. I avoid using alcohol or other drugs—especially illegal drugs—as a way of handling stressful situations or the problems in my life	2	1	0
3. I am careful not to drink alcohol when taking certain medicines (for example, medicine for sleeping, pain, colds, and allergies), or when pregnant	2	1	0
4. I read and follow the label directions when using prescribed and over-the-counter drugs	2	1	0
Alcohol and drugs score __________			
Eating habits			
1. I eat a variety of foods each day, such as fruits and vegetables, whole grain breads and cereals, lean meats, dairy products, dry peas and beans, and nuts and seeds	4	1	0
2. I limit the amount of fat, saturated fat, and cholesterol I eat (including fat in meats, eggs, butter, cream, shortenings, and organ meats such as liver)	2	1	0
3. I limit the amount of salt I eat by cooking with only small amounts, not adding salt at the table, and avoiding salty snacks	2	1	0
4. I avoid eating too much sugar (especially frequent snacks of sticky candy or soft drinks)	2	1	0
Eating habits score __________			
Exercise/fitness			
1. I maintain a desired weight, avoiding overweight and underweight	3	1	0
2. I do vigorous exercises for 15–30 minutes at least 3 times a week (such as running, swimming, or brisk walking)	3	1	0

3. I do exercises that enhance my muscle tone for 15–30 minutes at least 3 times a week (such as yoga or calisthenics)	2	1	0
4. I use part of my leisure time participating in individual, family, or team activities that increase my level of fitness (such as gardening, bowling, golf, or baseball)	2	1	0

Exercise/fitness score ___________

Stress control

1. I have a job or other work that I enjoy	2	1	0
2. I find it easy to relax and express my feelings freely	2	1	0
3. I recognize early, and prepare for, events or situations likely to be stressful for me	2	1	0
4. I have close friends, relatives, or others whom I can talk to about personal matters and call on for help when needed	2	1	0
5. I participate in group activities (such as church and community organizations) or hobbies that I enjoy	2	1	0

Stress control score ___________

Safety

1. I wear a seat belt while riding in a car	2	1	0
2. I avoid driving while under the influence of alcohol and other drugs	2	1	0
3. I obey traffic rules and the speed limit when driving	2	1	0
4. I am careful when using potentially harmful products or substances (such as household cleanser, poisons, and electrical devices)	2	1	0
5. I avoid smoking in bed	2	1	0

Safety score ___________

What your scores mean to YOU:

Scores of 9 and 10—Excellent! Your answers show that you are aware of the importance of this area to your health. More importantly, you are putting your knowledge to work for you by practicing good health habits. As long as you continue to do so, this area should not pose a serious health risk. In addition, you are probably setting a good example for your family and friends to follow. Since you got a very high score on this part of the test, you may want to consider other areas where your scores indicate room for improvement.

Scores of 6 to 8—Your health practices in this area are good, but there is room for improvement. Look again at the items you answered with a "Sometimes" or "Almost never." What changes can you make to improve your score? Even a small change can often help you achieve better health.

Scores of 3 to 5—Your health risks are showing! Would you like more information about the risks you are facing and about why it is important for you to change these behaviors? Perhaps you need help in deciding how to make the changes you desire. In either case, this book can help you.

Scores of 0 to 2—Obviously, you were concerned enough about your health to take the test, but your answers show that you may be taking serious and unnecessary risks with your health. Perhaps you are not aware of the risks and what to do about them. You can easily get the information and help you need to improve, if you wish. The next step is up to you.

or buckle your seatbelt without guidance from us. Nor will we deal with addiction to alcohol or other drugs; people with these problems usually need more individualized and intensive help than can be offered in a book of this nature. What we will zero in on are three important aspects of lifestyle that pertain to everybody, and for which there are general guidelines you can apply to yourself; they are exercise, nutrition, and stress.

Why have lifestyle factors assumed such a dominant role in causing disease and premature death? There are probably several reasons: One is that people live longer now that infectious diseases are under control and chronic diseases have more time to develop in people. The other major reason is that we have made some changes in our living habits that have had a negative impact on health.

Now let's look at how some aspects of our lifestyle have changed since the early part of this century.

Less exercise now

A century ago, Americans put a much greater amount of physical effort into their occupations than they do now. This can be seen in Figure 1.2 which demonstrates that work which used to be carried out mostly by humans and animals is now accomplished mainly by machines.

This tendency to decrease energy expenditure is also evident in household tasks as is shown in Figure 1.3. These observations also

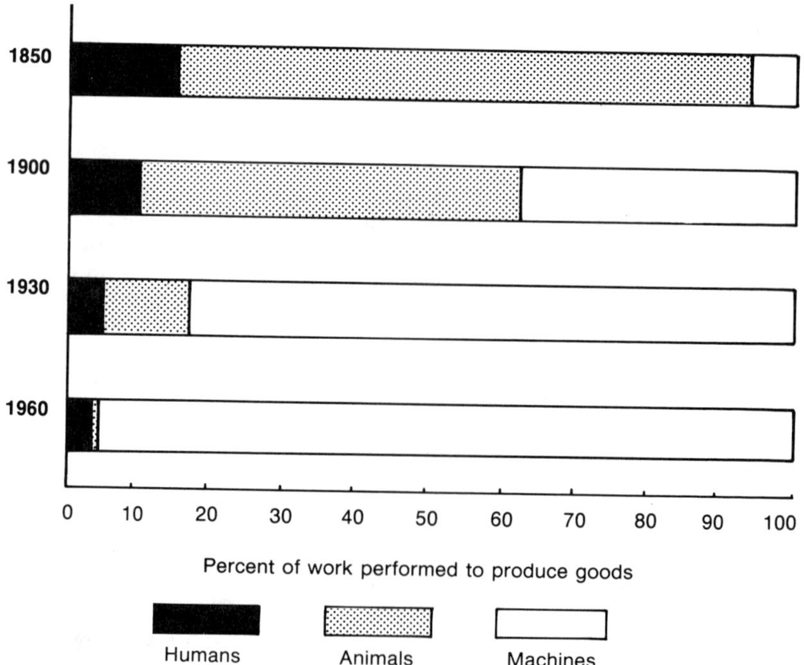

Figure 1.2 Changes in work performers during the past century. Dark bars, by humans; light bars, by animals; white bars, by machines.

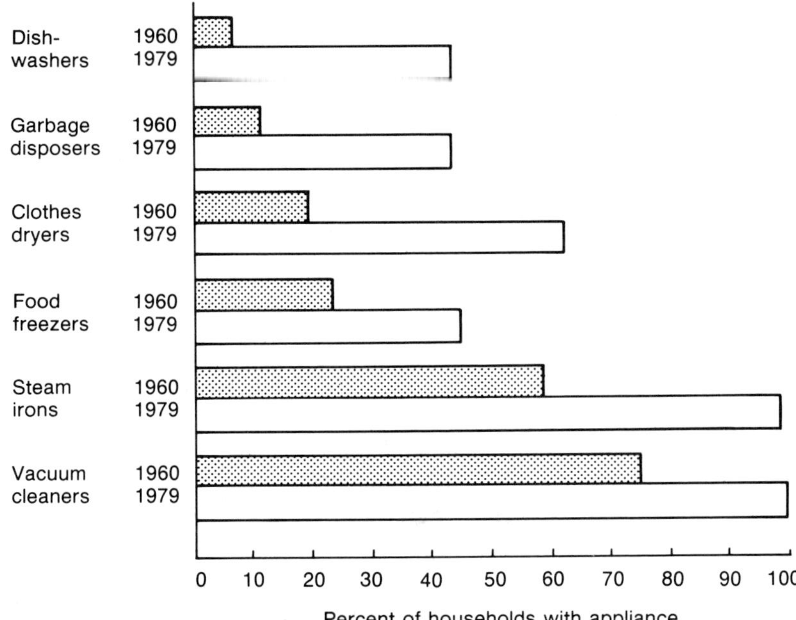

Figure 1.3   Increase in number of homes using labor-saving-devices. The graph shows what percentage of households had the different appliances.

suggest that there should be more time and energy available for recreational pursuits.

Travel also requires much less human energy expenditure now. In 1920 there was one automobile for every 13 Americans; in 1930 one for every 11 Americans; and in 1970 one for every 2 Americans. On the other hand, other figures suggest that one segment of the population is still interested in using their own power for transportation: In 1940 there were 1.3 million bicycles sold in the United States, but in 1973 fifteen million were purchased (Allen, 1975).

Different diets now

We can also compare changes in eating habits.

One important aspect of food is its energy value. According to the United States Department of Agriculture, the number of **kcalories** that have been available per person per day in this country has not changed much since the first part of the century. Although there have been minor fluctuations, the level of energy intake in the early 1980s was 98% of what it was in 1910 (Figure 1.4). Since Americans are eating about as many kcalories now but exercising less, you might expect overweight to be a problem. That is, in fact, the case; this issue will come up repeatedly in later chapters.

Another way in which food intake can be compared is the composition of the diet. Although foods as produced by nature have not

Kcalorie (kilocalorie or kcal, usually called "calorie" in the popular press): The unit of heat used to measure the energy value of a food; one kcalorie is the amount of heat needed to raise the temperature of one kilogram of water by 1° Celsius.

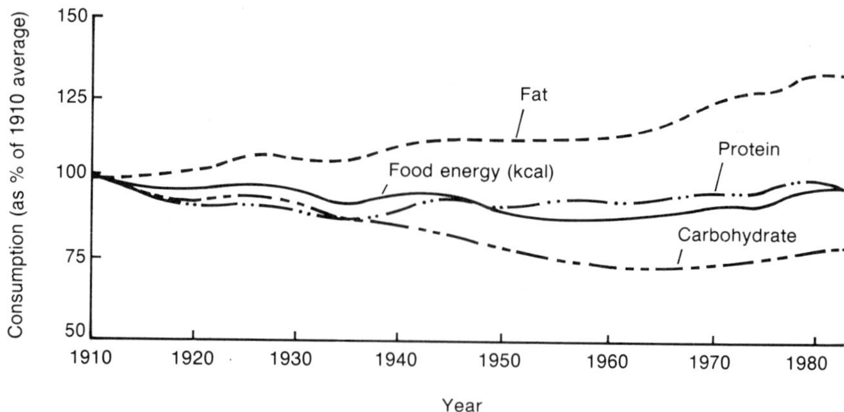

Figure 1.4   Trends in food and nutrient consumption from 1910 to 1982.

changed in composition from then until now—a fresh carrot in 1910 and a fresh carrot now have very similar levels of nutrients—the composition of the total diet has changed considerably. One reason for this change is that contemporary Americans tend to consume less unprocessed foods and rely increasingly on highly processed items.

Overall, we consume less carbohydrate than we used to (Figure 1.4). Even though we have increased our consumption of concentrated sugars, we have also dramatically decreased our intake of starch from grains and vegetables and of natural sugar from fruit, so that our net carbohydrate intake has dropped substantially.

On the other hand, overall intake of fats has increased significantly from 1910 to 1980. Most of that rise is due to increasing consumption of fats of plant origin, such as corn and soybean oils.

Daily total protein intake is now about the same as in 1910, but the source of this nutrient has changed. Formerly, plants and animals each provided about half of the protein consumed, but animal sources currently furnish a much larger proportion.

More stress now?

We have much less information on the role of stress in people's lives 75 years ago as compared with today. That is because the *concept* of stress is a fairly modern invention; therefore we do not have much historical data on it.

Dr. Hans Selye, a pioneer in the study of stress, defined stress as "the nonspecific response of the body to any demand made upon it." Stressors may be everyday events that tax us either physically or mentally (such as an upcoming exam, coming down with a cold, or mowing the lawn on a hot day), or they may be larger, more life-shaping events (such as getting married, deciding to change your occupation, being in a serious accident, or taking a long trip). Both unpleasant and pleasant events can cause stress. A certain amount of stress actually has a beneficial effect (*eustress*); but the concern for many people today is that the amount of stress they experience has become so great as to cause them *distress*.

We don't know for sure whether people are exposed to more stress now than before, but it may be that people who "live in the fast lane" pack more experiences—including stressful ones—into a given time span. One psychologist has suggested that our current lifestyles may produce a continual or background level of stress so high that when even minor stressors are added, we feel severely distressed. Another factor is that today many people have a much more tenuous support system than people had before; for example, those who live in communities of strangers far away from their extended families have fewer people close by who are ready to help them deal with their distresses.

Some of these changes in lifestyles are among the factors that researchers have found to be associated with increasing risk of chronic disease. Knowing which living habits are potentially dangerous can help motivate people to change. They also need to be aware that time is of considerable importance; the next section explains why.

Sooner Is Better

The sooner a person begins to improve his or her living habits, the better off that person will be. It is clear that prevention, not treatment, is the preferred approach to most of our current health problems.

One reason for this is that if people wait until the development of obvious illness, it may be too late; one-third to one-half of heart attack victims don't survive the first twenty-four hours. Also, when chronic diseases are present, they may impose limitations on a person's activities; even aggressive rehabilitation programs may not be able to restore full functioning. And from a financial perspective, it can be more expensive to cure or arrest a disease than to prevent it in the first place.

Many of the chronic diseases and disabilities which plague our middle-aged and older Americans have their beginnings early in life. Although a heart attack may occur at age 50, for example, the underlying disease probably began during childhood. Therefore prevention, to be most effective, must begin in young people.

Examine All Your Habits

It is also important to keep in mind that many of our most serious diseases such as heart disease and cancer probably are **multicausal (or multifactorial) diseases**; that is, there is no single risk factor which explains all or even a majority of cases. Risk factors can have an additive effect: if a person has one, he is more likely to develop the disease than someone who does not have any, but a person with two risk factors has a still greater chance of developing the disease.

Multicausal (or multifactorial) disease: An illness caused by several factors simultaneously.

Sometimes there are mitigating factors. For example, smoking is a risk factor for heart disease. Yet we all have heard of someone who smoked most of his life, is now over eighty years of age, and has never had any indication of heart disease. This does not prove that smoking is not a causative factor.

Rather, if we accept the concept of multicausal diseases, it indicates that this person had other things going for him. He may have been fortunate enough to have inherited the tendency toward long life, or he may have had healthy exercise and nutrition habits. In addition, a given risk factor may have less—or more—influence on one person's health than another's.

But since you have no way of knowing what genetic safeguards you may possess, or to what extent a bad health habit may undermine a good one, it is smart to try to develop all the good health habits you can.

For all of these reasons, it pays to adopt as many healthy living habits as early in life as possible. But making changes in established habits is not an easy thing to accomplish; permanent changes are in order, not just quick two-week exercise programs or diets that are promptly discontinued to return to old habits.

How can people make these permanent changes? We have probably all tried to reform ourselves in one way or another at some time, but have failed to make the new behavior habitual. How can we increase our chances of success in making lifestyle changes? That is what the next chapter will address.

Changing Behavior Successfully

2

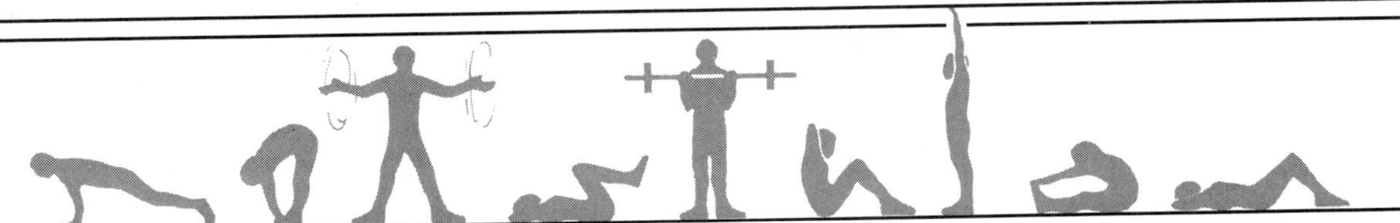

Outline

Have you ever had the experience of going on a weight-loss diet and, several weeks later, weighing more than when you started the diet? Or have you ever firmly resolved to "get in shape," only to hurt so much the day after the first workout that slothful inactivity took over again? Have you ever told yourself that you're not going to get uptight when you have to do another report in front of a class, but find yourself completely unnerved before your next presentation?

All of the above are common examples of attempted behavior changes that didn't work. You can see why it is difficult to form new habits when you consider how long we have practiced our old behaviors—months, years, or even all our lives. Therefore, simply saying to ourselves, "I'm not going to overeat anymore," or, "I am not going to get nervous when I do my next report," is not sufficient for successfully overcoming an entrenched habit.

Fortunately, there is an area of expertise that has much to contribute toward helping people change behavior, and that is the science of psychology. Behavioral psychologists have developed a process called behavior modification which has worked for all sorts of habit changes.

Behavior modification has been used by educators to help children change undesirable classroom behaviors; by parents to improve their children's behavior at home; and by mental health workers in the treatment of certain neurotic and psychotic behaviors. Within recent years it has been widely applied in health care settings as well. For example, many overweight people have learned to use behavior modification to control their food intake and thereby lose weight; others have used it to stop smoking, increase exercise, lower their dietary fat intake, and reduce many other troublesome behaviors. Because behavior modification is so useful for changing firmly set behaviors, we will discuss it here to help you make health habit changes.

One of the advantages of behavior modification is that once you learn the steps of the process and the concepts that underlie it, you can design your own programs. You do not need to have the help of a psychologist to use it, although the process is widely used by professionals as well.

In the past, some misinformed people have suggested that behavior modification is a sinister practice in which a therapist forces his or her own standards and values on others. Knowing that you can set up your own program should dispel any such concerns you may have had; even when used by responsible professionals for treatment, the first step is for the therapist and client to arrive at a mutually satisfactory agreement regarding the goals and methods to be used.

In this chapter we will give a brief introductory outline of the process, followed by an explanation of each step. At several points in the book, we will refer back to this chapter as we discuss specific applications of behavior modification. Therefore, if you are looking for more examples of this process in action, be assured that there are more ahead. This material provides an important background for what comes later.

With that as introduction, let's move directly to a brief listing of the steps in behavior modification:

1. Set your goal, for example, to achieve a particular level of fitness, or to lose a certain amount of weight.
*2. Record what your behavior is now in that area.
*3. Evaluate why you practice those behaviors.
4. Make a plan for change.
5. Implement it.
6. Monitor your progress.

Now for a more detailed discussion of each step.

---

*Sometimes steps 2 and 3 are combined.

Set Your Goal

We presume that people who are using this book want to improve their health. However, each individual will have different specific ideas about what would constitute better health for himself or herself.

For one person—let's call her Lisa—an important goal might be to decrease the amount of fat in her diet. She has learned that a high fat diet is a risk factor for both cardiovascular disease and cancer, and she thinks it possible that her typical intake might be higher than the recommended limit of 30 percent of kcalories from fat. Initially, she decides to set a goal of lowering her fat consumption to 30 percent. (Later, after she has discovered from the next step that her current fat intake is 41 percent of kcalories, she decides that a more reasonable goal would be 35 percent.)

Another person—John—might believe that he should quit smoking. He has known for a long time that there is a long list of health reasons to quit, but recently when he burned a hole in a new shirt with some stray cigarette ash, and on the same day overheard a very attractive woman in one of his classes comment that he smelled disgustingly of smoke, he suddenly decided to quit (a decision he had reached about ten times before). He decided to "go cold turkey," because most of his unsuccessful attempts had been to quit by gradually cutting down.

Note the characteristics of these objectives: they move in the direction of better health; they are as specific as possible; and they seem reasonable for the individuals involved. Try to build these features into objectives you design for yourself.

Although you might identify with one or both of the examples here, don't feel limited by them. Your objectives should relate to your own individual needs. Lisa and John just provide illustrations; your goals will probably be different, and tailor-made for you.

Record Current Behavior

Once you have established your goal, you need to look at what your current habits are in the aspect of living that your goal involves. Let's look at how Lisa and John might do this.

Lisa needs to make a record of her diet—what she eats, and how much of it—for several typical days. Since she knows her eating patterns vary considerably from weekdays to weekend days, she decides to record three weekdays and two weekend days. She tries to eat as normally as possible so the record will provide a true picture.

Lisa finds that peanuts are her favorite snack; she ate them eight times in the five days she recorded. Chocolate chip cookies hold second place, with five occasions.

After she has finished recording her intake for all five days, she uses the diet evaluation technique as described in the dietary assessment chapter for determining what percentage of her kcalories come from fat. (This is what influenced her to adjust her original goal somewhat.) She also scans the fat contents of the individual foods she ate to see which contributed the highest amounts of fat. She identifies butter, peanuts, and chocolate chip cookies as three culprits in her diet.

John makes a record as well. In order to remind himself to keep it, he wraps the piece of paper around his cigarette pack, uses a rubber band to hold it there, and tucks a short pencil under the band. He, too, tries to practice and record his usual habits, being careful not to let the recordkeeping influence his smoking behavior.

Evaluate Why You Practice Those Behaviors

In order to get to the upcoming step of planning how to change a habit, it is important first to analyze your record to find out (insofar as possible) what causes and maintains the behavior.

Lisa, for example, looks over her diet record to see whether the occasions on which she uses a lot of butter have anything in common. She finds that she uses most of the butter on baked potatoes and bagels. In other words, the mere presence of potatoes and bagels is an occasion for using butter.

Cue: An antecedent factor that sets the stage for a particular response.

The factors that promote Lisa's consistent use of the high fat items, potatoes and bagels, for example, are what psychologists call **cues** (or antecedents or discriminative stimuli). Cues can be quite diverse; they can be any factors that are part of our environment such as place, time, smell, sight, preceding activity, or people who are present. They can also be internal states such as moods.

But the cues Lisa has identified are not the only influences that lead her to the behavioral response of eating excessive butter, peanuts, and chocolate chip cookies. Certainly, one reason she eats these items again and again is simply because she likes them. The benefit—in this case the sensory pleasure she gets from eating these things—psychologists call a **positive reinforcer**.

Positive reinforcer: Something that occurs as the result of a response, making it more likely that the response will happen again.

A positive reinforcer is defined as an event or thing that is added to a situation following a response and that acts to strengthen the response. Lisa experiences a good feeling after eating butter, peanuts, and cookies, and this makes it more likely that she will eat these foods again.

However, there are more benefits for Lisa in eating these foods than the sensory pleasure she gets from them. She does most of her snacking while she is studying, and she uses the snacks as a periodic break; they relieve boredom and tension. Lisa's feelings of boredom and tension are called negative reinforcers. A **negative reinforcer** is defined as an event or thing which acts to strengthen a response if it disappears or decreases following the response. Lisa's consumption of butter, peanuts, and cookies is strengthened not only because it makes her feel good but also because it makes her feel less bored and tense. Note that Lisa's feelings of boredom and tension can function as cues as well as consequences. When Lisa feels bored or tense she has a snack, which, in turn, reduces her boredom or tension.

Negative reinforcer: Something that disappears or lessens as the result of a response, making it more likely that the response will happen again.

Both positive and negative reinforcers are strengthening consequences because they make it more likely that the behavior they follow will be repeated. The cues and the strengthening consequences are equally important in assuring that the behavior will happen again.

Now let's think about John for a moment. He has also been listing the cues that trigger his cigarette smoking. Drinking coffee, studying, watching TV, seeing somebody else smoking, and visiting with friends seem to be strong cues for him. John also knows that smoking has powerful strengthening consequences for him. He has figured out that his smoking is positively reinforced because it makes him feel more mature. The big negative reinforcement is that it is a relief from anxiety.

John also knows that there are distinctly unpleasant consequences of smoking. Burning holes in clothes and smelling of smoke are two that were already mentioned. Others are stained teeth and hands, and having to deal with dirty ashtrays and furniture scars. These are instances of something unpleasant appearing as a result of a behavior; such factors are weakening consequences, because they make it less likely that the response they follow will be repeated. Apparently these weakening consequences of smoking have not been powerful enough to overcome the strengthening consequences.

Many everyday behaviors are determined by cues and also by strengthening or weakening consequences. Psychologists call such behavior operant behavior. The behavior occurs in a specific setting and "operates" on the environment to produce a consequence which then functions to strengthen or weaken the behavior.

Many of our habits are examples of this type of behavior. In other words, our behaviors are not isolated events unconnected to anything else; rather, a given behavior is often part of a series of events, which, once it starts, is likely to go through to completion just as it has many times in the past. Because of this, it is usually easier to effect behavior change by changing the cues than by changing the behavior while all the cues are still there, coaxing you to continue the old habit.

Just as it will be useful for you to be aware of the cues that trigger the behaviors you are trying to change, it will also be useful to learn what strengthening consequences your habits have. In other words, what has been the reward for you when you have practiced those behaviors? Use the form in Self-check 2.1 for organizing and keeping track of your thoughts as they occur to you.

Then you're ready for the next step.

Once you are aware of the cues and consequences that influence your behavior, you are ready to plan your strategy for change. Three tools that behavioral psychologists have found to be useful are cue control, counterconditioning, and response cost.

Plan for Change

Self-check 2.1   Identifying the cues and consequences controlling your behavior

List the behaviors you want to change in the behavior column. Next list the cues for each behavior. In the columns on the right, note all the strengthening and weakening consequences for each behavior.

		Consequences	
Cues	Behavior	Strengthening	Weakening
1. 2. 3. 4. 5.		1. 2. 3. 4. 5.	1. 2. 3. 4. 5.
1. 2. 3. 4. 5.		1. 2. 3. 4. 5.	1. 2. 3. 4. 5.
1. 2. 3. 4. 5.		1. 2. 3. 4. 5.	1. 2. 3. 4. 5.
1. 2. 3. 4. 5.		1. 2. 3. 4. 5.	1. 2. 3. 4. 5.
1. 2. 3. 4. 5.		1. 2. 3. 4. 5.	1. 2. 3. 4. 5.
1. 2. 3. 4. 5.		1. 2. 3. 4. 5.	1. 2. 3. 4. 5.

Cue control

Cue control involves rearranging your environment so that the cues for the behaviors you want to weaken are *less* evident, and the cues for behaviors you want to strengthen are *more* evident.

For example, Lisa wants to cut down on her consumption of butter. She could, of course, simply avoid buying it and therefore it would not be there to tempt her. A more reasonable approach, since there is no need for her to give up butter entirely, would be for her to change her buying habits. Instead of buying a whole pound of butter each time she shops, she might buy just one stick (1/4 pound) to last her until the next time she goes. This would necessitate her using less on each potato and bagel to make the butter last. Another approach might be to cut down on the number of times she eats potatoes and bagels, which are cues for eating too much butter.

To rearrange his environment, John might remove all his ashtrays because he realizes they are cues to smoke. He could also stop drinking coffee, but he enjoys having a hot beverage at times during the day; therefore, he decides to try tea for a while which has never had an association with smoking for him. He goes through his entire list of cues in this way.

Sometimes there may be different alternatives for dealing with one cue. List them all; later you can always cross out those that don't suit you. For example, John smokes when he sees others smoking. He could choose to avoid his friends who smoke, but two of his very best friends are smokers. He might prefer instead to see less of them just at the start, and talk with them by phone during the early phase. If they happen to be part of a group he is with, he might sit so that they—and more importantly their cigarettes—are not directly in his line of vision.

Look over the cues you have listed in Self-check 2.1. Decide which ones you can control, and how you might do it.

Cue control: Changing cues in your environment in order to improve behavior.

Counterconditioning

When it is not possible to avoid, or otherwise control, a cue, it may be possible to learn a new response to it; this is called **counterconditioning**.

Lisa often reaches for a snack of peanuts or cookies when she wants a break from the boredom and tension of studying. As long as she is a student, she cannot avoid the many hours of studying—and the periodic sense of tedium that comes with it. But she could learn to respond in a different way when she feels she needs a break. In other words, she might try to learn a new way of reacting to the cues of boredom and tension. If she is studying at home, she might do stretching exercises for a break instead; it feels good, as well as relieving somewhat her boredom and tension, and has the fitness benefit of helping maintain flexibility. She could have a short phone conversation with a friend.

Counterconditioning: Learning a new response to a cue.

She might do a brief housekeeping task that needs to be done, thereby gaining a sense of accomplishment in addition to doing something other than eating. She might make a list with short suggestions on it before she starts to study; each time she needs a break, she can do the next thing on the list.

There are a couple of important matters to keep in mind when using counterconditioning. One is that it functions best if the new response to the cue makes the old one impossible. While Lisa is stretching, she cannot be eating cookies at the same time. However, if she tried reading a magazine as her new response, she could still eat cookies at the same time.

Another important point is that a new response has to have a payoff that is as good as the old one was, or a person will not stick with the new behavior. If the good feeling of a five-minute stretching routine isn't as satisfying as a couple of cookies, forget the stretching: it won't work. Finally, only Lisa herself can predict which new responses will have strengthening consequences potent enough to encourage her to repeat the new behavior until it replaces the old habit. This is because what turns one person on may turn another off.

If John is watching television and misses having something to do with his hands, he might overcome his smoking urge by doodling or doing a crossword puzzle; he decides to keep a puzzle book and a pencil on the table near his chair.

John finds that anxiety-provoking, or stressful situations, such as exams, are difficult to avoid. Counterconditioning can be used to reduce the stress caused by these situations. John can learn behaviors other than smoking to relieve his examination anxiety. In a later chapter we will discuss some procedures for reducing stress.

Response cost

Response cost: Losing an item of value as the result of practicing a certain behavior; a form of punishment.

Punishment: Something that happens as the result of a response, making it less likely that the response will be repeated.

Another means of changing behavior is called **response cost**. Response cost involves losing an item of personal value if you practice a "bad" behavior. Setting penalties for violations of rules and laws are examples of response costs.

Response cost is a form of **punishment**, having something bad happen to you for behaving in a certain way, with the result that the behavior is weakened. Although other forms of punishment are not usually as effective in changing behavior as positive and negative reinforcement are, response cost has been quite useful in helping people make certain health behavior changes. Both exercise and diet groups have used it by levying fines for missing sessions or regaining weight.

Smoking has some response costs inherent in it. The monetary cost of the cigarettes themselves is one example. John is aware of this cost but belittles it because it seems small on a day-to-day basis. It might become more impressive if he were to calculate the cost of all the cigarettes he smokes in a year.

Having done your preparation, it is now time to implement your plan—almost.

Now that you're poised at the starting line, there's one more thing to consider: when you begin practicing your new behaviors, you're bound to discover some consequences of them that you didn't anticipate. The unexpected pleasant consequences are likely to be surprises that you quickly accept and soon take for granted, whereas the unpleasant or aversive consequences may appear to be disproportionately large annoyances.

John found two nice surprises as a result of quitting smoking. One was that he began to have more endurance when he walked the hills and stairways of the campus; the other was that food began to taste better to him. Soon, he took these two substantial benefits for granted, but let the minor annoyance of missing his cigarette while he read the day's mail grate on him.

You should recognize from the outset that any change in behavior will present a "mixed bag" of consequences, but emphasizing the positive ones will help you to succeed.

A technique that can help get you over the hump at the beginning is to make a written contract with somebody concerning the new behavior you intend to practice. Write this contract *before* the day on which you start practicing your new behavior. Identify the new behavior you intend to practice, and make a commitment to report to your partner at stated intervals about how you are doing. Also specify the obligations of the partner. The act of putting your intentions in black and white heightens the sense of importance regarding the behavior change; and involving somebody else makes you feel responsible to another person as well as yourself. Make sure that each of you has a copy of the contract.

As you go along, you'll probably find that there is another nice payoff of having a contract with someone: your partner, knowing what you are trying to do, is very likely to compliment you for your efforts along the way. This is good positive reinforcement, and you need lots of it. Appreciate it whenever it's given. Getting reinforcement is so important that you should also deliberately give it to yourself in an ongoing way.

There are different ways to do this. One approach is through *positive self-talk*; that is, compliment yourself about what you are doing. When Lisa started using a smaller amount of butter on her bagel, she checked the nutrition label on the butter carton to find out by how much she was reducing her fat intake; this way she could appropriately congratulate herself. John would say to himself after enduring a social situation without smoking, "Good job on getting through that one! It had its tough moments, but you handled it. Keep it up!"

Another way to reward yourself is to promise yourself something that you have been wanting; if you adhere to the new behavior, keep the promise. Lisa told herself that if she cut down her intake of butter, peanuts, and cookies by half between now and Saturday, she could go to a particular movie that night. This helped motivate her. Your rewards to yourself need to be events or things that you know will please you; remember that reinforcers are very individual.

A final principle to keep in mind regarding the use of reinforcers is that the closer in time they occur to the performance of the new behavior, the greater the behavior-strengthening effect they will have. Positive self-talk satisfies this condition readily. Telling yourself immediately and frequently that you are succeeding enhances your chances of future success.

Monitor Your Progress

As time passes, it is important to monitor your progress because that tells you if your program is working. If it is, well and good; if not, change is in order.

In some instances, it doesn't take any fancy monitoring system to determine how well you are doing. It will be obvious whether John is successful at quitting smoking.

But whether Lisa is reaching her goal is harder to discern. Even if she has cut her butter, peanut, and cookie consumption by half, has this reduced her fat intake to her 35 percent goal? To find out, periodically (at least weekly at first) Lisa could keep a one-day dietary intake record and evaluate it as she did in the second step of this program. If the percentage of kcalories she gets from fat has decreased from her original 41 percent, she knows her efforts have been a success.

For people who haven't achieved their goals, perhaps eliminating more cues or using stronger reinforcement might be useful. They should reevaluate their program, and change it to make it more effective. That's one great benefit of behavior modification: it isn't a rigid, "canned" program that completely works or completely fails. It has many different aspects, each of which can be modified to make the program more effective. A behavior modification program is flexible.

It is also possible that a person who is having trouble with his or her program may be trying to do too much too soon. This is a matter that is specific to the individual and to the situation. For example, Lisa may find that she can't handle all the changes she has proposed in her diet at the same time; she may be more comfortable with beginning to reduce her cookie consumption only (because she thinks it will be the easiest to bring under control), and deal with the butter and peanuts later. It is important to go slowly when making dietary changes for the following reason: some people get such great pleasure from their favorite foods that if they try to reduce their intake too drastically in the beginning, they become uncomfortable, and even depressed, because it is difficult to make up for so much lost pleasure.

Now that we have covered the general guidelines for making successful behavior changes, let's focus on physiology and exercise. In Chapter 5, on exercise programs, psychologists will again have help to offer—about how to stick to an exercise program after you've begun.

The Basics of Exercise Physiology 3

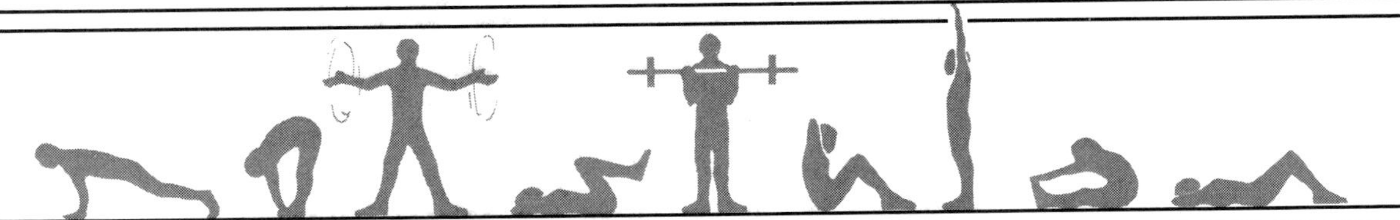

Outline

Early in the history of mankind, vigorous physical activity was an automatic and necessary part of daily life; people had to hunt and gather their food and flee their predators, or they would not survive. Later, people lived in groups for protection and had more reliable sources of food, and although many members of these communities still maintained high levels of physical activity, others no longer needed to expend as much effort in protecting themselves and providing for their existence. That was the start of a trend.

Leaping ahead to the present time, we find now that physical activity is largely a matter of choice. After all, most of us do not have to be on guard constantly for our physical safety. Technological advances enable machines to replace muscles in big and little ways: tractors, instead of men and animals, plow most farmers' fields; and we can change the television channel with a remote control instead of walking three steps to do it.

There is some risk in this trend toward inactivity, since if we use our **muscles** less and less, we gradually lose muscle power, fitness, and ultimately health. But the technological age need not be the death

Muscles: Organs which contract to produce movement.

23

knell for good health. Although our current situation no longer forces us to use our muscles, we can now choose *when* and *how* to use them . . . but not *whether* to use them, if we want to be healthy and fit.

Muscles must be used to maintain their function. If used vigorously enough, exercise actually increases the capabilities of muscles. These benefits are available to anybody who invests a relatively small amount of time and energy in a personalized exercise program.

In this chapter, we will introduce you to the most important piece of equipment needed for exercise—not skis, shoes, or weights, but something even more basic and versatile—your body. We'll begin by talking about the major systems involved in physical activity, how they function generally, and how they respond during exercise. This will provide you with a solid background for the chapters that follow, which will guide you in assessing your current physical fitness, and in setting up your own exercise program.

The Three Major Systems

You decide when to move your body. It's a conscious process initiated by your brain, which is linked by nerve cells to the muscles that control your body movement. Without this communication between your nervous system and your muscular system, you would be paralyzed. Because there are such vital interconnections between these two systems, they are often referred to together as the *neuromuscular* system.

Two other systems—your *respiratory* and *circulatory* systems—also play major roles during exercise. (You can't help but be keenly aware of your increased breathing and heart action when you're exercising.) These systems obtain and deliver the materials needed by your muscle cells for energy production, and carry away waste products.

Many other structures—such as bones, liver, and kidneys—play secondary roles, but we will not focus on them here. Rather, we will concentrate on the key systems we have identified. Although this chapter is structured to deal with these systems one at a time, you will find some overlap in the discussion because the system functions are so interrelated.

The neuromuscular system: where the action is!

Voluntary body movement occurs when an impulse from the thinking part of the brain—the cerebral cortex—travels through nerve cells that divide into many branches. Each *branch* of a nerve cell terminates on a *skeletal muscle cell*. The route the impulse takes is called the neuromuscular pathway. When an impulse reaches a muscle cell, energy is released, the cell contracts, and movement results. A nerve cell and the muscle cells it stimulates is called a **motor unit**, the functional unit of the neuromuscular system (Figure 3.1).

Muscle cells—which are also called **muscle fibers**—differ considerably in length. Some may be many centimeters in length, but even

Motor unit: A nerve cell and the muscle cells excited by all of the nerve cell branches.

Muscle cell or muscle fiber: The basic structural unit of a muscle.

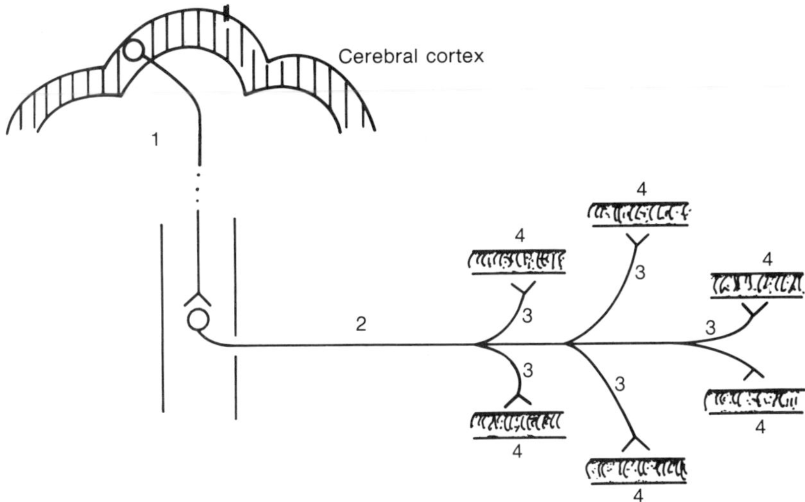

Figure 3.1   The neuromuscular pathway and a motor unit. To produce movement, an impulse travels from a nerve cell in the cerebral cortex of the brain (1), to a nerve cell lower in the brain or spinal cord (2), to its nerve branches (3), to muscle fibers (4). A motor unit comprises 2, 3, and 4.

the largest fibers are less than 0.1 millimeter in diameter. Muscle fibers are cylindrical in shape.

Within each muscle cell are hundreds of smaller structures called **myofibrils**. Myofibrils contain a high concentration of *contractile proteins* and *proteins which regulate contraction*. It is the action of these contractile and regulatory proteins which bring about movement. Figure 3.2 is a diagram of a muscle, muscle bundles, muscle fibers, and myofibrils.

Myofibril: Contractile and regulatory proteins of a muscle cell.

The only way to increase these proteins—which results in an increase in the number of myofibrils—is to do physically stressful work or exercise; the stress is the stimulus for the muscle cell to make more protein. When people lift weights or otherwise exercise to increase their muscle mass and strength, they increase the *number* of myofibrils within each fiber. When people lose muscle mass because of physical inactivity, *myofibrils are lost*.

There is some evidence that training may increase fiber (cell) number due to a "splitting" of existing fibers. This matter is a subject of some controversy. However, the gain or loss of myofibrils with training or detraining, respectively, is well documented.

A muscle is a group of muscle fibers that are bound together and work together in contraction to develop **muscle tension**. The muscles used in physical activity are called *skeletal muscles* because they are attached at their ends to the bones of the skeleton. When these muscles contract they *pull* on bones. Skeletal muscles make up nearly half of your body weight. Figure 3.3 identifies the major skeletal muscles. Two other types of muscle contract and generate tension but do not pull

Muscle tension: The force developed by muscle in contraction.

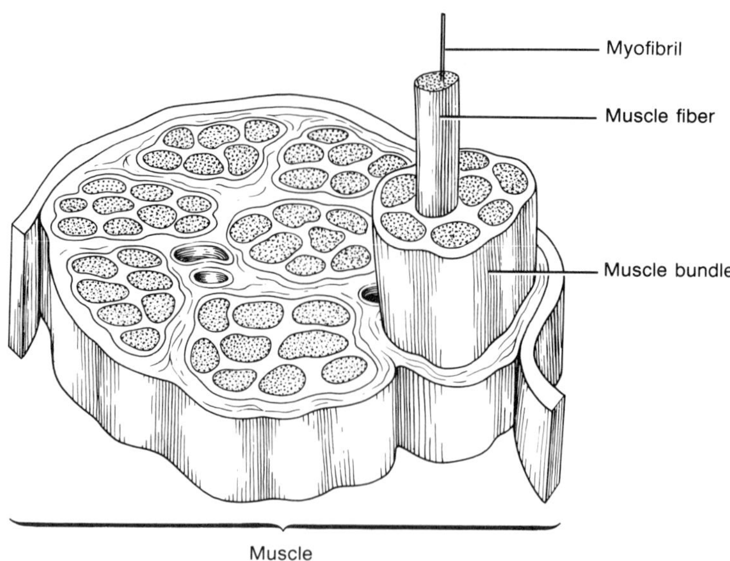

Figure 3.2   The relationships among whole muscle, muscle bundles, muscle fibers, and myofibrils.

on bones. *Cardiac muscle* in contraction propels blood from the heart's chambers and *smooth muscle* in contraction typically constricts blood and respiratory vessels and walls of digestive organs.

Skeletal muscle contractions are of three different types. If a muscle shortens when it contracts (as happens when the biceps shortens and moves the hand toward the shoulder) this process is called an *isotonic contraction*. If a muscle contracts but does not change in length (such as the muscles that are active when you clasp your hands and attempt to pull them apart), this process is an *isometric contraction*. A contraction in which the muscle lengthens (such as a lengthening contraction of the biceps which occurs when lowering a hand-held weight from the shoulder) is an *eccentric contraction*.

There is another factor that is needed for movement besides nerve impulses and muscle fibers, and that is *energy*. Muscle fibers are their own energy factories: each cell contains energy sources (energy substrate) which it metabolizes (chemically changes) to produce energy. The energy sources are *carbohydrate, fat,* and *protein*. The process of metabolizing these foodstuffs may occur in the body of the muscle cell (cytoplasm) or in a specialized cell structure, the *mitochondrion*. It is in the mitochondrion that aerobic metabolism occurs.

Carbohydrates and fats are the most important energy sources, in that their **metabolism** usually accounts for 85 to 95% of the energy used by the body. Protein is only a relatively minor energy source, but it has other unique and important functions. Nonetheless, it is available as a back-up energy source if carbohydrate and fat metabolism cannot keep pace with the body's energy needs (as might occur in a 100-mile bicycle race, for example).

Metabolism: Collective term for all of the chemical changes that take place in a living organism.

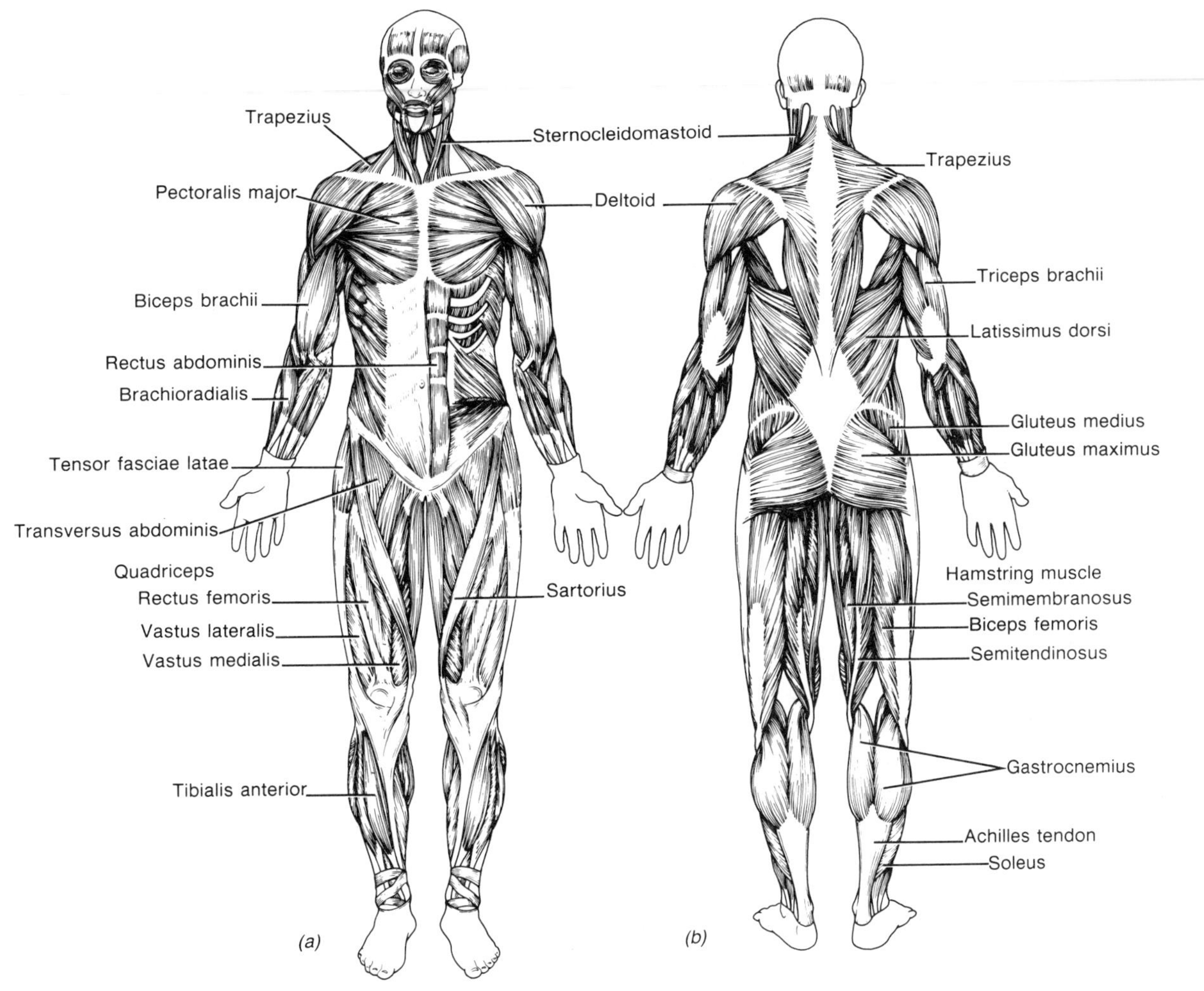

Figure 3.3   The major skeletal muscles. (a) Front view. (b) Rear view.

Can your muscle cells run out of carbohydrate and fat to metabolize? If you had to rely entirely on the carbohydrate and fat that are *stored in the muscle cells*, you would be in trouble, because they are present in only limited amounts at any given time. However, carbohydrate and fat from elsewhere in the body can be delivered to the cells to support continued energy production. For example, a human liver typically stores approximately 85 grams (3 ounces) of carbohydrate in the form of **glycogen** (sometimes called animal starch); glycogen can be broken down into **glucose** (a simpler carbohydrate form), released from the liver, and transported via the bloodstream to the cells that need it. Similarly, fat cells that are concentrated in fat-storage tissue (adipose tissue) can release their stored fat molecules to be delivered in the blood to muscle cells.

Glycogen: A form of starch that is stored in animal liver and muscle.

Glucose: A simple sugar used for energy by living organisms.

Table 3.1 gives you an idea of how much carbohydrate and fat are available in a human body. You can see that the body has much more stored fat than carbohydrate. Since, overall, we produce energy in roughly equal amounts from fat and carbohydrate, it is carbohydrate that will be used up first. However, most people's daily activities don't come close to exhausting their carbohydrate stores; this is more likely to happen to endurance athletes who exercise intensely and continuously for hours at a time. When a marathon runner experiences "hitting the wall" after about 20 miles, he or she has probably seriously depleted carbohydrate at that point.

Eating a high carbohydrate diet can help a person store higher-than-normal levels of carbohydrate, which can help increase endurance. This will be discussed later, in Chapter 10.

Now let's focus on the respiratory and cardiovascular systems which deliver materials to muscles and make continued exercise possible.

The respiratory system

Respiratory system: The organs that bring oxygen into an animal system and eliminate carbon dioxide.

Your **respiratory system** carries out the breathing process which brings atmospheric air (21% of which is oxygen) into your body and eliminates excess CO_2. Oxygen is needed by the body's cells for aerobic energy production. (Aerobic means "with air"; we will discuss aerobic energy production later in this chapter.)

Here, we want to emphasize that aerobic energy production is necessary not only for physical activity, but also for maintaining the continuous functions of the systems that keep us alive, such as the beating of the heart, the activity of the nervous system, and breathing itself. Therefore, if we don't get a steady supply of oxygen, we die within a few minutes. If a person's respiratory system becomes blocked, by a piece of steak, for example, this is a life-threatening situation.

At the same time that the respiratory system brings oxygen (O_2) into the body, it also removes excess carbon dioxide (CO_2). This gas is a

Table 3.1	Amounts and energy values of stored carbohydrate and fat for a 154-pound man (70 kg)	
	Amount (grams)	Energy value[a] (kcal)
Carbohydrate		
Glucose	20	80
Glycogen		
In liver	85	340
In skeletal muscles	350	1,400
Total carbohydrate	455	1,820
Fat[b]		
Total fat	10,500	94,500

[a]Carbohydrates yield 4 kcal/gram. Fats yield 9 kcal/gram.
[b]Fat is assumed to be 15 percent of body weight.

by-product of aerobic energy production. The structure of the respiratory system is shown in Figure 3.4.

The respiratory system consists in part of **airways** (mostly bronchi and bronchioles), a branching series of narrower and narrower channels through which air moves on its way to the small lung sacs where exchange of gases with blood occurs. The smaller airways have smooth muscle in their walls which allows them to constrict (get smaller in diameter) or relax (get larger). For unknown reasons, some people are afflicted with periods of inappropriate constriction which cause increased resistance to airflow through the channels. These people have the condition called *asthma*. During an asthmatic attack, a person has to breathe very hard in order to get enough oxygen to the lung sacs and to remove enough carbon dioxide which has been returned to the lungs.

The location at which oxygen actually enters the body's interior and carbon dioxide leaves it, is the lung exchange tissue. This **lung tissue** contains millions of tiny air sacs called *alveoli* (singular, alveolus) that cluster like grapes at the ends of the smallest airways (see Figure 3.4).

Alveoli have such thin and moist membranes around them that gases can easily dissolve into the fluid and move freely through the membranes. Immediately adjacent to the alveoli are microscopic blood vessels called *capillaries*, which also have thin membranes that allow the passage of dissolved gases.

Blood entering lung capillaries is lower in oxygen and higher in carbon dioxide than the air in the alveoli. These differences cause oxygen molecules to move from the alveoli into the capillaries. At the

Airways: The tubes of the respiratory system through which gases pass.

Lung tissue: A system of air sacs (alveoli), which exchange oxygen and carbon dioxide with lung capillaries.

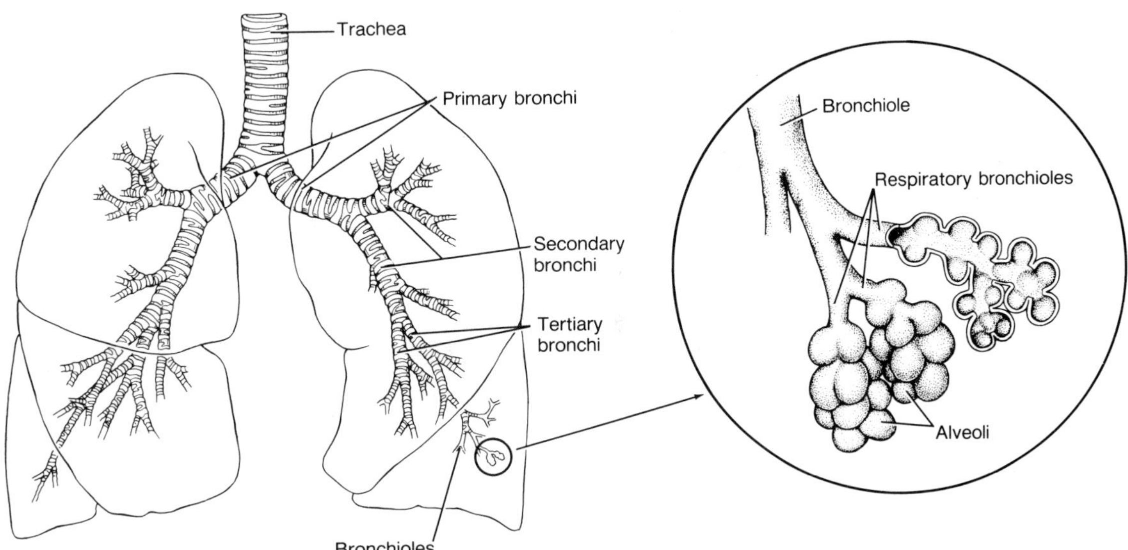

Figure 3.4 Important features of the respiratory system.

Exchange of gases: Passage of oxygen into and carbon dioxide out of the body.

same time, carbon dioxide molecules move from the capillaries into the alveoli. This **exchange of gases** (Figure 3.5) is due to *diffusion* (movement of gas from high to low concentration) which can occur rapidly over short distances.

Muscles are also part of this system. When you inhale, inspiratory muscles (including the diaphragm) contract, expanding the chest cavity and creating a partial vacuum in the lungs; air rushes in to equalize the pressure. To breathe out, expiratory muscles (including some of the muscles of the rib cage) contract, which makes the chest cavity smaller, squeezing gases from lung tissue through the airways into the atmosphere. Your breathing *ventilates* the alveoli (keeps O_2 and CO_2 concentrations constant so exchange with blood can continue).

Your breathing *rate* (number/minute) and *depth* (volume of air/ breath) are largely automatically controlled by the nonthinking part of your brain, based on your body's needs. During exercise, the amount of O_2 and CO_2 that must be exchanged goes up dramatically—and therefore so does your breathing rate and depth. Table 3.2 is an example of this. *Minute ventilation*—the amount of air (in liters) either inspired or expired each minute—increases as the product of the breathing rate and depth (volume). Aerobic training tends to cause a decrease in minute ventilation at submaximal exercise intensity.

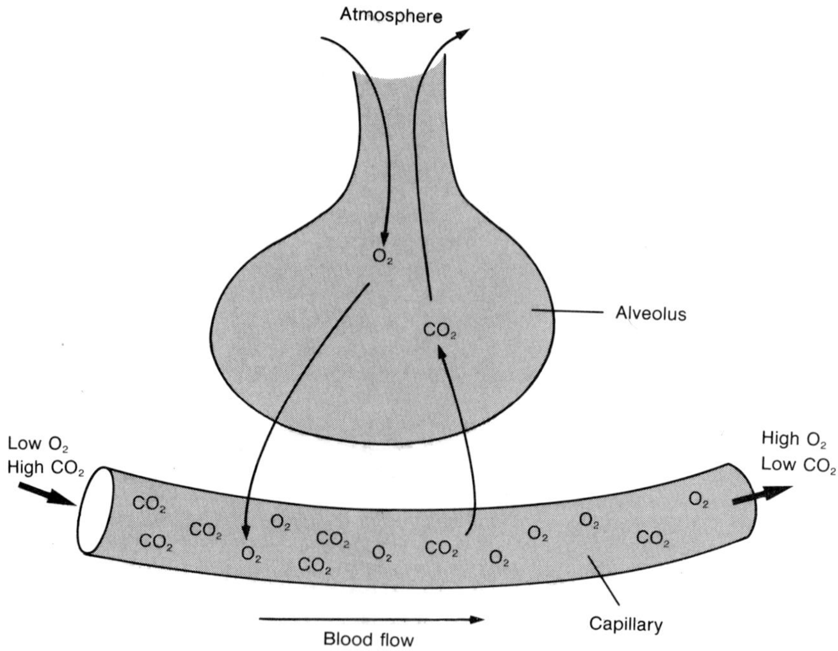

Figure 3.5   Exchange of gases. The body is supplied with oxygen (O_2) by the movement of oxygen molecules from the alveoli, through the membranes of the alveoli, and then through the membranes of the capillaries into the blood within the capillaries. Carbon dioxide (CO_2) leaves the body by the reverse route.

Table 3.2 An example of the effect of exercise on breathing

	Breathing rate (breaths/min)	Breathing depth volume (liters)	Minute ventilation (liters/min)
Rest	12.0	0.5	6.0
Moderate exercise	25.0	1.5	37.5
Maximal exercise	40.0	2.5	100.0

The circulatory system

The circulatory or cardiovascular system is the body's transport system. It carries not only gases, but also nutrients and waste products as well. This system consists of the heart and a continuous network of blood vessels in which the body's 5 to 6 liters of blood (the blood volume) cycles repeatedly. (A liter is 1.06 quarts.)

Your *heart* is the pump that keeps blood moving through your circulatory system. It is composed of cardiac muscle that normally contracts 50 to 90 times per minute when the body is at rest. Within the heart are four chambers, called the right and left atrium and the right and left ventricle, which expel blood each time the heart beats. The chambers fill with blood during the relaxation phase of the cardiac cycle.

The vessels that enter and leave your heart are few in number but large in size, since the body's whole blood supply is channeled through them. Vessels going away from the heart are called *arteries*. They branch repeatedly into *arterioles*, which finally branch into an intricate network of tiny blood vessels called *capillaries*. (We have already mentioned the capillaries of the lungs: capillaries serve every other organ of the body as well.) It is through the capillary membranes that oxygen, nutrients, and waste products pass between the body's blood supply and body cells. Continuing the circuit back toward the heart, the capillaries thicken, enlarge, and converge into *venules*, which join into larger and larger *veins* that eventually empty blood back into the heart.

The two circuits There are two loops of vessels through which the body's blood is continuously routed. One loop—the *pulmonary circuit*—circles between the heart and the lungs to allow for the exchange of gases between the blood and outside air. The other—the *systemic circuit*—connects the heart to all organs of the body for the pickup and delivery of substances needed for metabolism and for the removal of waste products (Figure 3.6).

Each circuit is powered by a different side of the heart, the pulmonary, by the right ventricle and the systemic, by the left ventricle. You could liken the route blood takes through these loops to a "figure 8" that is continuously being redrawn; the heart is positioned in the middle, where the loops meet. Blood courses through both circuits simultaneously and continuously throughout your lifetime.

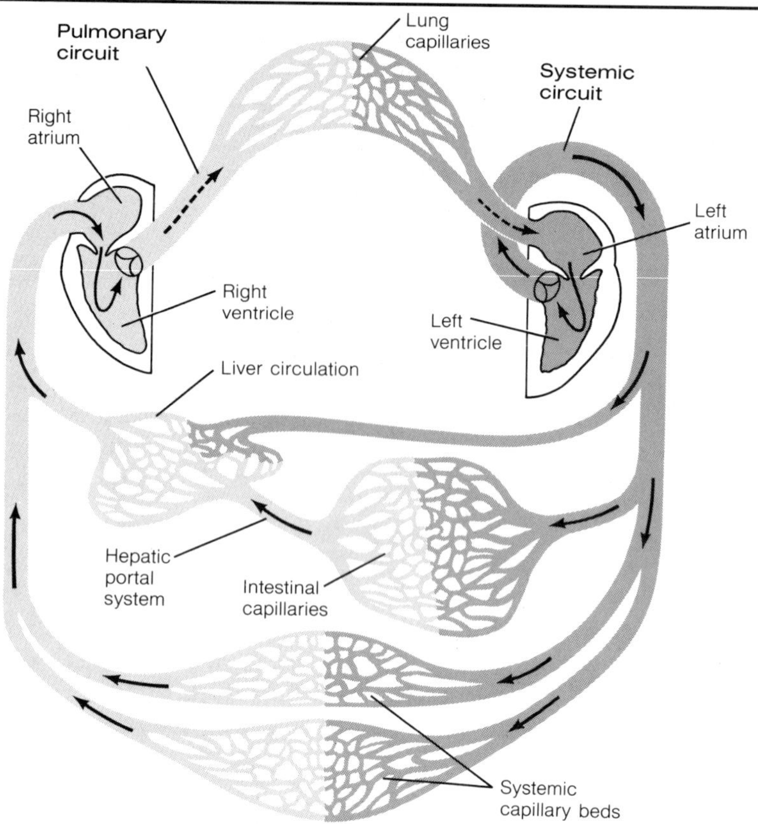

Figure 3.6 A schematic representation of the cardiovascular system. The right heart chambers propel blood into the pulmonary circuit (dashed arrows) and the left heart chambers propel blood into the systemic circuit (solid arrows).

The blood Now let's focus on the *blood* itself for a moment. More than 90% of the blood is water; the remainder is dissolved substances, several of which have been mentioned already—oxygen, carbon dioxide, and nutrients. There are also substances in blood called *carriers*, which are materials that bind with other compounds in the blood.

Hemoglobin: A blood protein that binds oxygen.

One important carrier in blood is **hemoglobin**, an iron-containing protein to which oxygen binds in red blood cells. Under normal conditions, 99% of the oxygen in blood is bound by hemoglobin; only 1% is present as free gas. Therefore, the concentration of hemoglobin in the blood influences how much oxygen can be carried to all the body's organs.

Women normally have slightly lower hemoglobin concentrations in their blood then men do, so their maximal oxygen-carrying capacity is somewhat lower. Since the amount of oxygen available to exercising muscles is directly related to the amount of energy the muscles can produce, for women this lower capacity can be a disadvantage in performance of aerobic events.

People who have **anemia**, a lower-than-normal level of red blood cells and/or hemoglobin, are also limited in the amount of oxygen their blood can deliver to various organs for energy production. Someone who is anemic will not be able to perform as well during activity as he or she would with adequate levels of hemoglobin.

Cardiac output   Now let's get back to the movement of the blood through your body. During every heartbeat each ventricle pumps about half of the volume of blood within it into your pulmonary and systemic circuits; this is referred to as the **stroke volume** and amounts to about 80 milliliters at rest. Since your heart is an elastic muscle that can stretch, it has the capacity to increase its stroke volume. The number of times your heart beats per minute (*heart rate*) can also change. The product of the stroke volume times the heart rate gives the *cardiac output*, the amount of blood that each ventricle expels into the pulmonary and systemic circuits each minute. During exercise, a special part of your nervous system that functions automatically and involuntarily—the **sympathetic nervous system**—causes your heart to greatly increase its cardiac output so it can deliver more oxygen and nutrients to muscle cells.

Let's look at how a person's cardiac output at rest might compare with cardiac output during exercise. The numbers used here are just examples; although they are typical values there is a large range as to what is normal. Note that physiologists use the metric system, and therefore measure blood volumes in milliliters (ml) or liters ($=1000$ ml); there are approximately 30 ml in a fluid ounce.

	At rest	During exercise
Stroke volume (ml)	80	120
$\times$ Heart rate (beats/min)	$\times$ 70	$\times$ 190
Cardiac output (ml/min)	5,600	22,800

In this example, exercise caused cardiac output to rise to about four times the rest value (22,800 ml/min compared with 5,600 ml/min). The effect varies with the intensity of the exercise.

Another way in which the cardiovascular system helps keep muscle cells supplied with what they need is by controlling blood distribution. For example, at rest the kidney receives about 1.5 liters of blood flow per minute, while your entire skeletal muscle system receives only about 1.0 liter/min of blood flow. However, in strenuous exercise the kidney may receive only 0.3 liters/min, and active muscle as much as 15.0 to 20.0 liters/min.

How is this redistribution accomplished? To understand the mechanism, we need to look more closely at the structure of *arterioles*, the small blood vessels that connect the arteries to the capillaries. Arterioles contain smooth muscle in their walls. When this muscle contracts, it

Anemia: A condition associated with low levels of red blood cells and/or hemoglobin.

Stroke volume: The amount of blood (in ml) pumped from a ventricle of the heart in a single contraction.

Sympathetic nervous system: System that controls heart rate, the force of heart contractions, arteriole resistance, and vein capacity.

constricts the opening through the arterioles, and there is more re-sistance to blood flow. When this muscle relaxes the opening becomes larger (dilates) and there is less resistance to blood flow. The contraction and relaxation is controlled by centers in the brain which convey a message by way of the sympathetic nervous system to arteriolar smooth muscle, to constrict or dilate.

During exercise, sympathetic nerve activity to internal organs such as the kidney is increased; the kidney arterioles constrict; and blood is diverted (due to increased resistance to blood flow) to regions where there is less resistance. Active skeletal muscles and heart muscle, on the other hand, have minimal constrictor activity. Therefore, their ar-terioles are dilated and there is little resistance to blood flow. In this way, muscle blood flow increases as blood is diverted from constricted organs. This diversion of blood from other organs, coupled with the higher cardiac output described earlier, supplies active skeletal muscle and cardiac muscle with their greater needs during exercise.

Arterial blood pressure   Of course, in order for this mechanism of blood distribution to work, there has to be pressure that pushes the blood through the vessels. Just as you need a certain water pressure in your plumbing system in order for water to get to the kitchen and bathroom faucets, you need adequate blood pressure in your arteries to get blood to all regions of your body.

Pressure is created in the arterial system when the heart pumps blood into the arteries with each contraction. The pressure in the arterial system at any time varies with the amount of blood the heart pumps into the arteries (cardiac output) and the amount of blood that escapes through the arterioles (resistance vessels) into the capillaries.

The pressure in the arteries of the systemic circulation can be de-termined by using a *stethoscope* to detect sound and a *sphygmomano-meter* (an occluding cuff and a mercury column). Pressure is measured in millimeters of mercury (mmHg) (Figure 3.7). Pressure is measured both when the heart muscle is contracting and expelling blood (*systole*) and when it is relaxing (*diastole*). Therefore a blood pressure reading consists of two numbers, such as 120/80 mmHg.

The first number refers to the pressure in arteries when the heart is expelling a mass of blood (stroke volume) (**systolic pressure**), and the second number represents the lowest pressure attained between beats (**diastolic pressure**)—when blood is leaving the arterial system for dis-tribution to capillaries. Many health care providers regard the lower number as the one to watch most carefully; if it exceeds 90 mmHg at rest, it indicates borderline *hypertension* (high blood pressure). This may eventually damage the heart because the heart has to work harder when pumping against the higher diastolic pressure in the arteries.

Exercise and arterial pressure   When you start to perform a rhythmic exercise which involves a large mass of muscles, like running or cycling,

Systolic pressure: The maxi-mal pressure measured in a systemic artery during a heart beat.

Diastolic pressure: The min-imal pressure measured in a systemic artery during re-laxation after a heart beat.

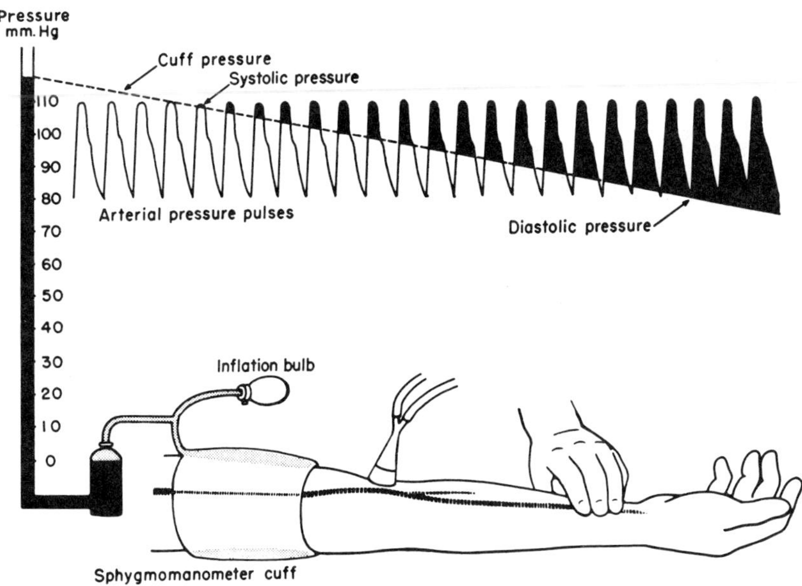

Figure 3.7 How arterial blood pressure is measured. The arterial pressure—which is commonly called the blood pressure—is measured by wrapping a sphygmomanometer cuff around the upper arm. A stethoscope is placed on the inner arm below the cuff in order to listen to the sounds in the artery of the arm. The cuff is then inflated by repeatedly squeezing the inflation bulb, raising the pressure in the cuff sufficiently to close off blood flow through the artery. The cuff pressure is then reduced slowly. Eventually, during a heart contraction (systole), the blood pressure is high enough to overcome the falling pressure in the cuff, and blood courses turbulently through the artery, making an intermittent thumping sound. The pressure at which the sound is first heard is recorded as the systolic pressure. With continued pressure reduction, the sound disappears. The pressure at which the sound completely disappears is recorded as the diastolic pressure.

your cardiac output increases, which makes your systolic pressure increase. However, the arterioles that control the blood flow to the muscles involved in the activity gradually relax (resistance to blood flow is reduced) as the exercise proceeds, so that a greater volume of blood can leave the arteries between beats and flow selectively into the capillaries that serve the exercising muscles. Since more blood escapes from the arteries between beats of the heart, diastolic pressure remains at resting level.

The above paragraph describes how blood pressure usually responds to exercise involving a large, active muscle mass contracting rhythmically, such as running, cycling, rowing, or swimming. However, a somewhat different effect occurs during activity using a limited amount of muscle mass, such as weightlifting, or holding a heavy suitcase. With the effort localized to fewer muscles, fewer muscle arterioles dilate, keeping muscle resistance to blood flow relatively high. While cardiac output is increased the failure of muscle resistance to decrease causes both systolic and diastolic pressure to increase. Extremely high arterial pressures may occur in a person lifting heavy weights.

This type of activity is often promoted in the popular press as a convenient way for people to exercise. However, it could have serious consequences, especially for those who already have high blood pressure. Other types of exercise do not generally carry this risk. We will say more about high blood pressure in the chapter on cardiovascular disease.

Cardiovascular effects of training   Aerobic training can produce the following changes from the pretraining state in cardiovascular function:

1. Reduction in resting heart rate
2. Increased rest stroke volume
3. Lower heart rate and higher stroke volume through a range of submaximal exercise loads (no change in cardiac output)
4. Maximal heart rate unchanged and maximal stroke volume increased (increased cardiac output)
5. Rest and exercise blood pressure slightly lower

Two Ways of Producing Energy

Aerobic metabolism: The process of completely utilizing carbohydrate, fat, and/or protein to produce energy and carbon dioxide and water as byproducts.

Anaerobic metabolism: The process of incompletely utilizing carbohydrate to produce energy and lactic acid as a byproduct.

Now we understand how the respiratory and cardiovascular systems can deliver more O_2, carbohydrate, fat, etc., to muscles in exercise. The next consideration is, how do muscle cells deal with these materials in supplying energy for muscle contractions?

Basically, your body produces most of the energy it needs by combining carbohydrate and fat with oxygen in a process called **aerobic metabolism**. There is also an auxiliary system called **anaerobic metabolism**, in which carbohydrate alone can provide brief surges of additional energy, which we will discuss later in this chapter.

Aerobic energy production

The cells of your body continuously produce energy aerobically, using oxygen taken in by the respiratory system and distributed by the circulatory system. When you are at rest, aerobic metabolism is the source of most of your energy. It also produces most of the energy you use when you walk, swim, cross-country ski, row, run a distance, or do any other rhythmic activity that you could sustain continuously for more than 15 minutes at a time. Such types of exercise are called aerobic activities.

The following chemical reactions describe what happens during aerobic metabolism within the mitochondria of the cells:

$$\left.\begin{array}{c}\text{Carbohydrate}\\\text{or}\\\text{fat}\\\text{or}\\\text{protein}\end{array}\right\} + \text{oxygen} + \text{ADP} + \text{P} \rightarrow \text{ATP} + CO_2 + \text{water} + \text{heat} \qquad (1)$$

This chemical reaction shows that carbohydrate, fat, or protein reacts with oxygen (aerobic reaction) by taking the energy from the nutrient and transferring it to a complex chemical compound called **adenosine diphosphate (ADP)**. Diphosphate means two phosphate atoms are attached to adenosine (adenosine$\cdot$P$\cdot$P). When energy is transferred from a foodstuff, it is bound between the second and third phosphate atoms (adenosine$\cdot$P$\cdot$P$\sim$P) and now the compound is called **adenosine triphosphate (ATP)**. The squiggly line between phosphates (P$\sim$P) indicates a high-energy bond. Only adenosine$\cdot$P$\cdot$P$\sim$P can be used to supply muscle directly with energy. Muscles store some readily available energy in this form, but the total supply amounts to no more than 5 kcalories, so it must constantly be supplied by reaction (1). Adenosine diphosphate (ADP) is *not* useful as an energy source.

As ATP is used by muscle cells when they contract, the following reaction occurs:

$$\text{Adenosine}\cdot\text{P}\cdot\text{P}\sim\text{P} \xrightarrow{\text{energy release}} \text{adenosine P}\cdot\text{P} + \text{P} \qquad (2)$$

To replace the ATP used, reaction (1) above must occur again. It should be apparent that intense exercise may severely tax the ability of the metabolic system to supply adequate ATP for muscle use.

Aerobic activities are done at such a pace that the body's respiratory and circulatory systems are able to provide enough oxygen to active muscle cells to metabolize nutrients and supply ATP to meet energy needs. If this pace is exceeded the necessary ATP must come from anaerobic metabolism.

It is possible to quantify your body's capacity for aerobic metabolism. This is done by measuring the largest volume of oxygen you can absorb into your lung capillary blood from your lung alveoli in one minute, while exercising vigorously—usually cycling or running. Special equipment such as that seen in Figure 3.8 is needed for making this determination.

This value—the largest volume of oxygen you can absorb in a minute—is called your maximal oxygen uptake ($\dot{V}_{O_2}$ max) and represents your *aerobic capacity* (or *maximal aerobic power*).

$\dot{V}_{O_2}$ max may be increased by aerobic training. Studies have reported increases ranging from 5 to 30%. The magnitude of the change depends on the $\dot{V}_{O_2}$ max at the beginning of training. The training effect (increased $\dot{V}_{O_2}$ max) is due to two main factors: (1) an increase in the

Adenosine diphosphate (ADP): The compound formed when energy is released from ATP and one phosphate group is split off.

Adenosine triphosphate (ATP): A high energy compound found in living cells; the immediate source of cell energy.

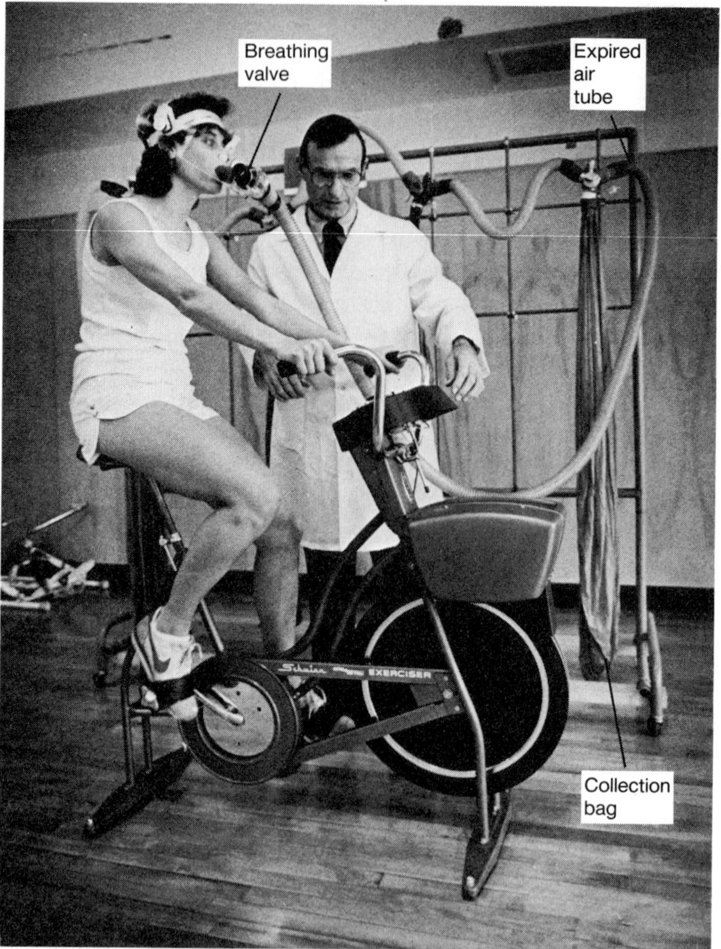

Figure 3.8   How maximal oxygen uptake ($\dot{V}_{O_2}$ max) is determined. $\dot{V}_{O_2}$ max is determined by collecting the air expired during a given number of minutes of strenuous physical activity as shown here. After the expired air is analyzed for oxygen and carbon dioxide contents, the volume of expired air is measured, and the amount of oxygen that was removed from the air—and therefore taken up by the body—can be calculated.

maximal cardiac output, and (2) an increase in the number of mitochondria in muscles. The mitochondria, which are found inside most cells, are where aerobic metabolism occurs. This additional aerobic machinery makes it possible for the muscle cells of a trained athlete to process more oxygen and produce more ATP.

There are occasions when it is not possible for the body to supply enough oxygen to meet energy needs aerobically; in other words, some activities are done at an energy demand exceeding 100% of $\dot{V}_{O_2}$ max. For example, in running a 100- or 200-meter sprint the rate of energy use greatly exceeds what can be supplied aerobically. In such situations anaerobic metabolism supplies additional energy.

Anaerobic energy production (glycolysis)

Sprinting in any sport, weight lifting, and running as fast as you can to catch a bus are all examples of activities for which anaerobic metabolism provides extra energy. The characteristic these activities share is that they demand a huge amount of energy in a very short period of time; anaerobic metabolism can provide the needed surge of energy over and above what the body can produce aerobically.

The only energy source that can be used for anaerobic metabolism is carbohydrate. We have already mentioned the two major forms of carbohydrate found in the body—blood glucose and the carbohydrate storage form, glycogen. Because glycogen is split into its constituent glucose molecules during anaerobic metabolism, this process is also called *glycolysis*.

Glycolysis does not require oxygen. That is why it can provide additional energy when aerobic metabolism is using all the oxygen that is available. Another difference between the two types of metabolism is that in glycolysis, carbohydrate is incompletely metabolized and a substance called *lactic acid* is produced. The accumulation of lactic acid in muscle cells is associated with fatigue and discomfort, so glycolysis is useful for only a few minutes at a time.

The process of glycolysis is summarized by the following chemical reaction:

$$\left. \begin{array}{c} \text{Glucose} \\ \text{or} \\ \text{glycogen (in muscle)} \end{array} \right\} + \text{ADP} + \text{P} \rightarrow \text{ATP} + \text{lactic acid} + \text{heat} \tag{3}$$

This brings to mind another difference between the two types of metabolism: glycolysis is not very efficient at regenerating ATP. In fact, aerobic metabolism produces 18 times more ATP from a given amount of carbohydrate.

What happens to the lactic acid after you stop your activity? Gradually, it is either aerobically metabolized to energy, carbon dioxide, and water, or it is converted back to glucose in the liver. You know from your own experience that after you have performed an all-out activity, you don't feel eager to move your muscles again for a while.

Thus far we have discussed the usefulness of glycolysis for high intensity activities, such as sprinting and weight lifting; but there are also other circumstances in which glycolysis acts as a booster system.

For example, some activities vary considerably in their intensity during the time you are doing them, so that you may need help from glycolysis intermittently. Tennis is one good example of this. When balls are consistently hit right to you during a game, you don't have to move much to return them; aerobic metabolism is adequate in this situation. But if you are at the back of the court and your opponent drops a shot just over the net, you will have to hustle if you want to get it; then you need glycolysis for a temporary lift to get to the net.

Many team sports—such as soccer, baseball, football, water polo, and volleyball—call for similar intermittent use of glycolysis. Such activities require a combination of aerobic and anaerobic metabolism.

You even use glycolysis briefly during true aerobic activity. Whenever you start an aerobic activity, you put an immediate demand for increased energy—and therefore for more oxygen—on your body. Even though your body has the capability of eventually meeting your energy needs for that activity aerobically, it takes a few minutes to "rev up" for the task. A more technical way of describing this is to say that during the first few minutes of an aerobic activity, the response of the respiratory and circulatory systems lags behind energy demand, and a large portion of the energy during the start-up phase must be supplied by glycolysis (anaerobically). This is the case every time you exert yourself above rest levels for any form of work or play.

After you have finished aerobic exercise and are at rest, you continue to breathe deeply for a few minutes and consume O_2 above rest needs. Some of this O_2 is used to metabolize the lactic acid that was produced in the first few minutes of exercise, before the O_2 consumed was sufficient to meet the energy need. In this early phase of exercise one incurs an **oxygen deficit** which calls for an **oxygen repayment** after exercise. Figure 3.9 illustrates this.

From these examples, you can see that there really is no form of exercise that involves only glycolysis (anaerobic metabolism) or only aerobic metabolism.

Oxygen deficit: Occurs at the onset of exercise when oxygen use does not keep pace with energy use.

Oxygen repayment: Occurs at the end of exercise; oxygen uptake remains elevated in order to replace ATP used while oxygen deficit was accumulating.

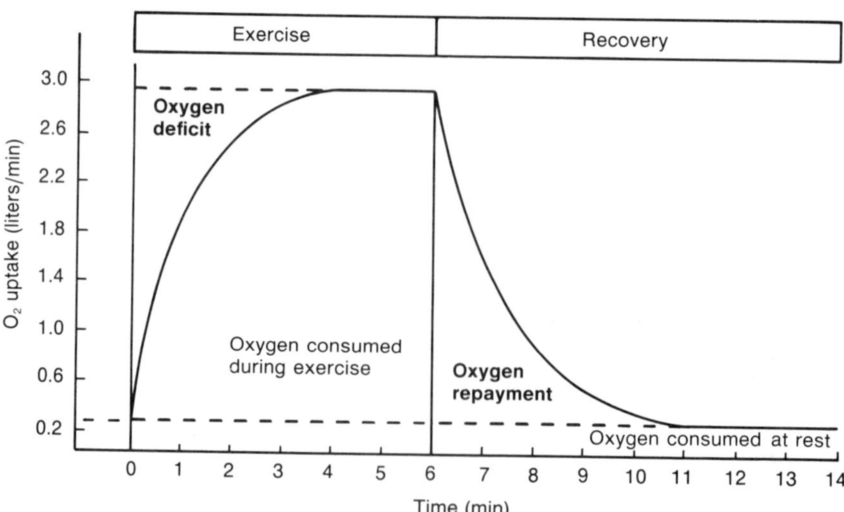

Figure 3.9   Oxygen deficit and repayment during aerobic activity. The oxygen requirement is 2.9 liters O_2/min. For the first 3 to 4 minutes, this requirement is not completely met by the O_2 consumed. During this time stored ATP and glycolysis with ATP formation must supply some of the required energy. After exercise is terminated (6 minutes), the energy requirement returns to the rest level. However, O_2 consumption only returns slowly to rest level because the ATP stores depleted in exercise must be restored and any lactic acid accumulated must be metabolized.

The effect of muscle fiber types

There is another factor that influences the ratio of aerobic to anaerobic metabolism that occurs during exercise, and that factor is the relative amounts of the two muscle fiber types in a person's body. Muscle cells can be categorized as either **fast twitch or slow twitch muscle fibers,** depending on the speed at which the proteins within them contract as the muscles are used.

Fast twitch and slow twitch muscle fibers: Muscle cells that are categorized according to the speed at which they contract.

When individual muscles in the average person are analyzed, it is apparent that there can be a larger proportion of one type over the other within a particular muscle; up to 80% of the fibers can be of one fiber type. Depending on which type of fibers predominate, the whole muscle is referred to as a fast twitch or slow twitch muscle, even though a *muscle is always a mixture of the two types.*

Muscles that help you maintain your posture—and any other muscles that are used for long-term efforts—are likely to contain more slow twitch fibers; these muscle cells produce their energy aerobically. On the other hand, fast twitch fibers generally dominate in muscles used for brief, intense activities such as high jumping and sprinting. Whereas some fast twitch muscle fibers specialize in anaerobic energy production, others use predominantly aerobic metabolism.

If *all* of the skeletal muscle cells of an average human are considered, there are about equal amounts of fast and slow twitch fibers, even though the distribution is different within a particular muscle (as discussed above).

But some people are far from average in this regard; their genetic heritage has equipped them with a much higher overall proportion of one type. In fact, when a variety of elite athletes were evaluated for their overall proportions of skeletal muscle types, some striking differences were seen: Some cross-country skiers and distance runners were found to have approximately 80% slow twitch muscle fibers, whereas some sprinters had as high as 80% fast twitch fibers.

You might wonder whether such athletes developed more of one type of fiber because they trained in particular sports, but this is not the case because you are born with your fast and slow twitch fibers already determined. Rather, these athletes probably gravitated to their particular sport because the proportion of fiber types already present enabled them to excel at those specific activities.

Finally, what does all this information about structures, functions, and energy metabolism have to do with improving your fitness? Essentially, it sets the stage for taking the next step, which is for you to evaluate how you measure up in regard to the three major criteria that physiologists use to assess fitness—endurance, strength, and flexibility. It also prepares you to determine how much energy you expend in any particular activity, or in a whole day. These are the challenges of the next chapter. And after you have read it and done the self-checks, you will know better what the objectives of your own exercise program should be.

Measuring Fitness and Physical Activity   4

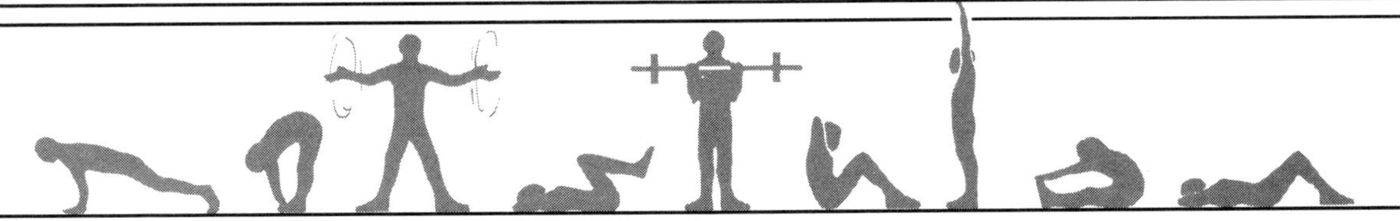

Outline

How do you think you measure up with regard to physical fitness and activity level?

Tim believes he must rate well. He plays basketball with a group of athletic friends for an hour three times each week; they play hard and are sweat-drenched and exhausted by the time they finish.

Ann feels good about her fitness now that she has been lifting weights for three months. She works out every other day on an exercise apparatus, and has increased the amount of weight and number of repetitions she can handle with every muscle group.

Jennifer has been doing daily calisthenic exercise using a video tape. For almost an hour each day, she puts herself through the series of bends and stretches that the entertainer featured in the video claims has maintained her enviable form.

Bob does not plan any physical activity for his spare time because he thinks he gets enough exercise by working 20 hours per week as a waiter. He is on his feet continuously while on the job; during part of that time he is carrying heavy trays of dishes and food.

Whose activity is providing the greatest benefit?

It is difficult to compare the activities of Tim, Ann, Jennifer, and Bob, because they affect different aspects of fitness. Tim's vigorous basketball playing has primarily been increasing and/or maintaining his aerobic capacity. Ann has been developing her muscular strength, whereas Jennifer is mainly improving her joint flexibility. Bob's job as a waiter has probably increased his strength somewhat, but not to the extent that Ann's progressive weight-lifting program has done for her. However, Bob may be at the head of the pack in terms of the amount of energy he expends each week.

This chapter will give you some tools for evaluating your fitness and activity level. There are also other, more sophisticated means of testing fitness and physical activity level than those we have included here; however, we have chosen these particular methods because they are reasonably valid tests and because the testing equipment needed is likely to be available in a typical gymnasium or athletic department.

Why is strength important? For one thing, a person with a reasonable level of muscular strength is more likely to maintain an efficient postural alignment with less fatigue and pain. Secondly, fewer injuries are to be expected if there is more muscle bulk and strength. Thirdly, it may be less fatiguing to lift and carry weights. A given weight or load (for example: lifting a child) represents a smaller percentage of maximum for a strong person as compared to a weaker person. It follows then that the stronger person should experience less fatigue at the end of the day. Finally, strength is an important ingredient of performance in most sports.

How Strong Are You?

There are many different kinds of tests that measure strength. You can test strength when the body is stationary (*static* strength), or in motion (*dynamic* strength). You can test for force that is instantaneously delivered (muscular *power*), or sustained for a period of time (muscular *endurance*). And you can test different muscle groups for each of these various capacities.

Another important factor in any discussion of strength is whether it should be measured in absolute or relative terms. That is, should a person who weighs 150 pounds be expected to lift the same amount of (absolute) weight as one who weighs 275 pounds, or is it more reasonable to expect a person to lift a load proportional to his or her own body weight?

Absolute strength: Total force exerted.

Absolute strength—expressed as total force exerted in kilograms or pounds—is pertinent in many situations. For example, people who respond to fire alarms need to be able to drag hoses of a given weight, or sometimes carry people. And for those who engage in such sports as football, baseball, and bowling, absolute strength is an important component of performance.

Relative strength is determined by dividing absolute strength by body weight. Relative strength separates out the effect of body size on strength, since large people generally have larger muscles and tend to be stronger in an absolute sense than smaller people. In some situations, relative strength is more important than absolute strength, such as when you are hanging onto an overturned boat, or pulling yourself out of a swimming pool. In wrestling competition, the fact that there are weight classes of participants indicates that the contest is one of relative strength. Another sport in which relative strength is more important than absolute strength is gymnastics.

In this chapter we will describe a number of tests that will help you measure your absolute and/or relative strength, power, and muscular endurance. Although some of these tests require special equipment, we have also included some that can be done without sophisticated equipment.

Static strength

Static (or isometric) strength is the force that can be exerted by a group of muscles instantaneously and with very little movement. A person cracking a walnut shell is using static strength.

A common way of measuring static grip strength is to squeeze a grip dynamometer as hard as you can. Figure 4.1 illustrates the use of this

Relative strength: Force exerted per unit of body weight.

Static (or isometric) strength: The force a group of muscles can exert instantaneously and with very little movement.

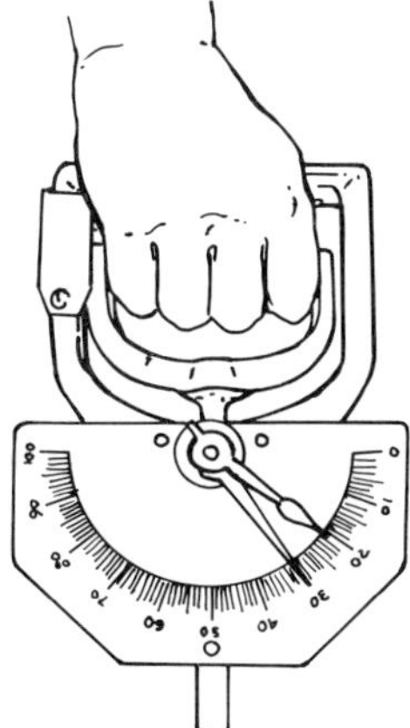

Figure 4.1   Measuring static grip strength using a grip dynamometer. First the dynamometer is adjusted for the size of the hand. Then the grip is squeezed as hard as possible. The instrument is held away from the body when force is applied. Usually, the test is performed twice with each hand. A brief rest should occur between trials. The total of the better score for each hand is then determined.

Table 4.1   Static grip strength: absolute and relative[a]

		Percentile	Scores by age[b]					
			17	18	19	20–24	25–29	30–34
(a) Absolute values[b]	**Males**	90	111	117	118	122	123	124
		80	105	106	113	115	115	115
		70	99	101	109	110	110	110
		60	93	98	104	105	107	106
		50	89	96	101	102	103	102
		40	85	93	98	99	100	98
		30	81	90	94	94	95	95
		20	76	86	90	89	90	90
		10	70	81	84	80	81	82
		Mean	91.5	97.1	102.0	102.9	103.6	103.4
	Females	90	61	59	63	61	67	65
		80	54	55	59	57	62	60
		70	50	52	54	53	57	57
		60	47	49	50	50	53	53
		50	44	46	48	48	49	49
		40	42	43	46	45	48	47
		30	39	39	42	42	46	44
		20	36	36	39	38	43	41
		10	31	31	36	34	37	36
		Mean	46.8	47.1	49.9	48.7	52.2	51.5
(b) Relative values[c]	**Males**	90	1.62	1.62	1.75	1.73	1.72	1.64
		80	1.48	1.50	1.54	1.59	1.54	1.52
		70	1.44	1.47	1.44	1.53	1.47	1.45
		60	1.39	1.44	1.36	1.45	1.40	1.39
		50	1.35	1.37	1.33	1.39	1.35	1.33
		40	1.28	1.33	1.29	1.32	1.28	1.29
		30	1.21	1.31	1.24	1.26	1.20	1.24
		20	1.16	1.22	1.17	1.18	1.12	1.18
		10	1.01	1.16	1.12	1.08	1.01	1.10
		Mean	1.32	1.37	1.37	1.39	1.34	1.35
	Females	90	1.12	1.02	1.10	1.04	1.12	1.05
		80	1.02	.95	1.04	.97	1.02	1.00
		70	.96	.90	.94	.91	.97	.94
		60	.89	.82	.85	.86	.91	.89
		50	.83	.78	.80	.81	.86	.83
		40	.78	.72	.77	.77	.82	.78
		30	.71	.69	.74	.72	.75	.72
		20	.66	.65	.69	.68	.68	.66
		10	.52	.58	.64	.61	.61	.60
		Mean	.83	.79	.85	.82	.86	.83

[a]Two trials were given with each hand using an adjustable dynamometer; the better score with the right was added to the better score with the left.
[b]Scores are the sum of right and left grip strength in kilograms.
[c]Scores represent the sum of right and left grip strength relative to body weight in kg per kg body weight.

equipment. Table 4.1*a* shows the distribution of performance ratings for hundreds of men and women of different ages who were evaluated for grip strength on an absolute basis. The figures in Table 4.1*b*, on the other hand, represent their grip strengths calculated relative to body weight.

Another way of measuring static strength of your arms is to use a device such as the arm dynamometer pictured in Figure 4.2. The data in Table 4.2*a* reflect the distribution of absolute strength for people of various ages using this equipment; Table 4.2*b* gives values for relative strength. Notice that most of the values for relative arm strength of women are below 1.0 on both Tables 4.1*b* and 4.2*b*. This means that most women cannot lift their own body weight by their arms.

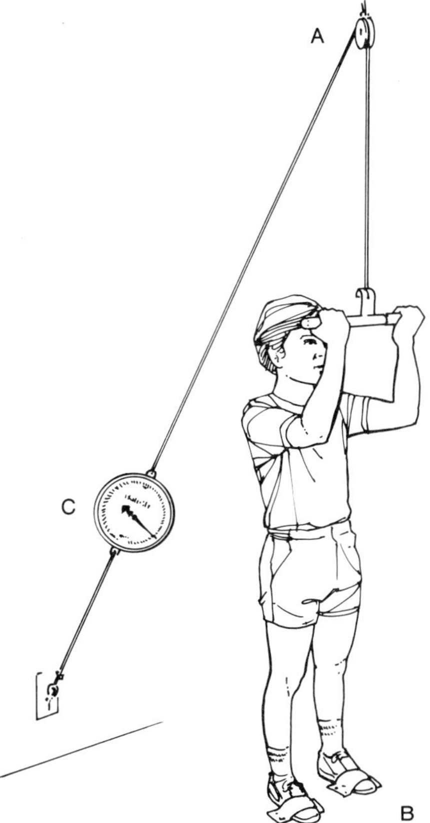

Figure 4.2 Measuring static arm strength. The subject places his/her feet in toe straps on the base (B) and grasps a bar with an undergrip (knuckles away from face) and with the hands shoulder-width apart. The cable connecting the bar to the dynamometer (C) passes over a pulley (A). The cable length is adjusted so that the angle of the elbow is 90 degrees and the upper arms are parallel to the floor. The person then exerts maximum pull on the bar gradually, without jerking, and the score is read from the dynamometer. Usually two trials are given with a brief rest in between. The better effort constitutes the score.

Table 4.2 Static arm strength: absolute and relative

			Scores by age[a]					
		Percentile	17	18	19	20–24	25–29	30–34
(a) Absolute values[a]	**Males**	90	100	106	115	113	112	114
		80	93	98	104	105	107	107
		70	88	94	98	100	103	101
		60	86	90	93	95	98	97
		50	83	87	90	92	94	94
		40	81	84	87	90	90	90
		30	78	80	84	86	87	86
		20	72	74	81	81	82	81
		10	62	65	77	72	75	74
		Mean	83.4	88.0	94.1	93.4	94.8	94.3
	Females	90	57	55	56	57	60	60
		80	52	53	54	54	55	55
		70	49	51	52	51	52	53
		60	47	49	49	49	49	51
		50	46	47	47	47	47	49
		40	44	45	45	45	46	47
		30	43	44	43	43	44	45
		20	39	40	40	40	42	42
		10	33	36	36	37	38	36
		Mean	47.0	47.3	47.7	47.9	48.9	49.2
(b) Relative values[b]	**Males**	90	1.44	1.52	1.57	1.52	1.49	1.48
		80	1.38	1.45	1.48	1.44	1.44	1.41
		70	1.32	1.38	1.40	1.38	1.36	1.34
		60	1.27	1.30	1.32	1.33	1.29	1.28
		50	1.23	1.20	1.27	1.26	1.23	1.21
		40	1.20	1.18	1.16	1.21	1.17	1.18
		30	1.10	1.13	1.11	1.15	1.10	1.13
		20	1.03	1.04	1.05	1.10	1.01	1.06
		10	.90	1.00	.94	.98	.92	.95
		Mean	1.20	1.24	1.26	1.26	1.22	1.23
	Females	90	1.04	1.00	.97	.96	1.00	1.00
		80	.98	.95	.90	.91	.92	.94
		70	.92	.88	.86	.86	.88	.90
		60	.90	.83	.84	.83	.85	.85
		50	.85	.82	.82	.82	.82	.82
		40	.82	.76	.77	.79	.78	.78
		30	.74	.71	.74	.75	.74	.75
		20	.70	.66	.71	.69	.71	.68
		10	.63	.63	.64	.61	.65	.61
		Mean	.84	.80	.80	.81	.82	.82

[a]Scores represent arm strength in kilograms.

[b]Scores represent arm strength in kg/kg body weight.

A test for static strength of the back is shown in Figure 4.3; performance scores for men are shown in Table 4.3. Unfortunately, we know of no such values established for women.

In general, absolute strength usually increases with age until a person reaches age 20 to 30, and then plateaus; it usually begins to decline sometime during age 50 to 60. Relative strength, the value calculated on a force-per-pound basis, increases until age 20 to 30 and declines steadily thereafter because people usually gain weight as they age.

The average man has greater muscular strength than the average woman in both absolute and relative terms. In large part, this may be due to the fact that in men, approximately 45% of body weight is muscle, whereas women's bodies are approximately 36% muscle. Perhaps this difference has a hormonal basis, but it probably also has a societal component: males usually receive more encouragement to develop their strength capacities than women do (Wells, 1985).

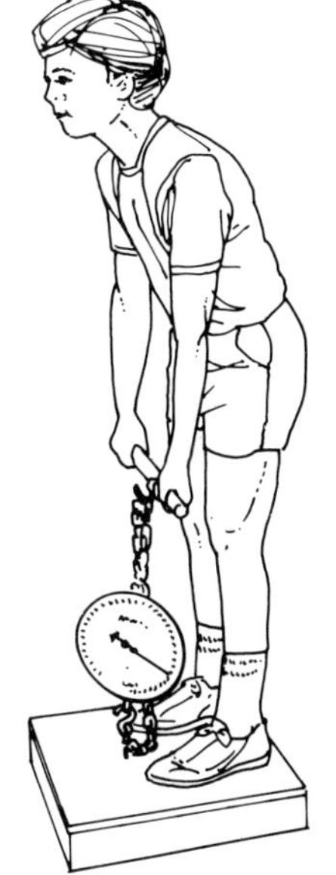

Figure 4.3   Measuring static strength of the back. The feet are positioned below the bar as illustrated. With the person to be tested standing upright with arms and fingers extended downward, the chain is adjusted so the bar is just at the fingertips. The person then grasps the bar firmly with one hand overgrip (knuckles facing away from the body) and the other hand undergrip (knuckles facing the body) and pulls upward with as much force as possible. The score is read on the dial and, after a brief rest, the test is repeated. The better of the two scores is used.

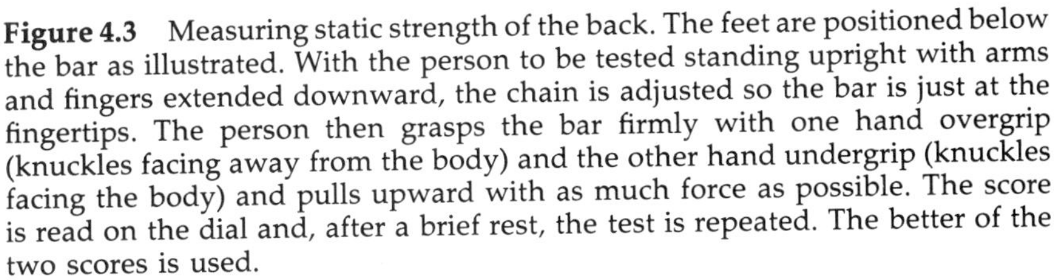

Table 4.3   Static strength of the back for men (absolute and relative)

Percentile	Strength	
	Absolute (lb)	Relative[a]
90	485	3.03
80	459	2.82
70	436	2.66
60	418	2.52
50	402	2.39
40	386	2.28
30	370	2.19
20	353	2.09
10	332	1.94

[a]Relative strength is measured in lb per lb of body weight.

Dynamic muscular endurance

Dynamic muscular endurance involves repeated muscular effort over a range of motion. Push-ups, pull-ups (or "chin-ups"), and sit-ups, illustrated in Figure 4.4, measure dynamic muscular endurance. On the other hand, how long you are able to hold yourself suspended from a horizontal bar is not an example of dynamic muscular endurance because there is no movement around a joint.

By their nature, these are relative tests in that you are moving your own body weight when you do them. As we pointed out earlier, most women are unable to lift their body weight by their arms; for them, pull-ups are impossible. This is reflected in the fact that there are little data for women's pull-ups. Since part of the body weight is supported by the feet during push-ups many women can do either the regular or modified version.

Table 4.4 gives standards for push-ups, pull-ups, and sit-ups.

Dynamic muscular endurance: Repeated muscular effort over a range of motion around a particular joint.

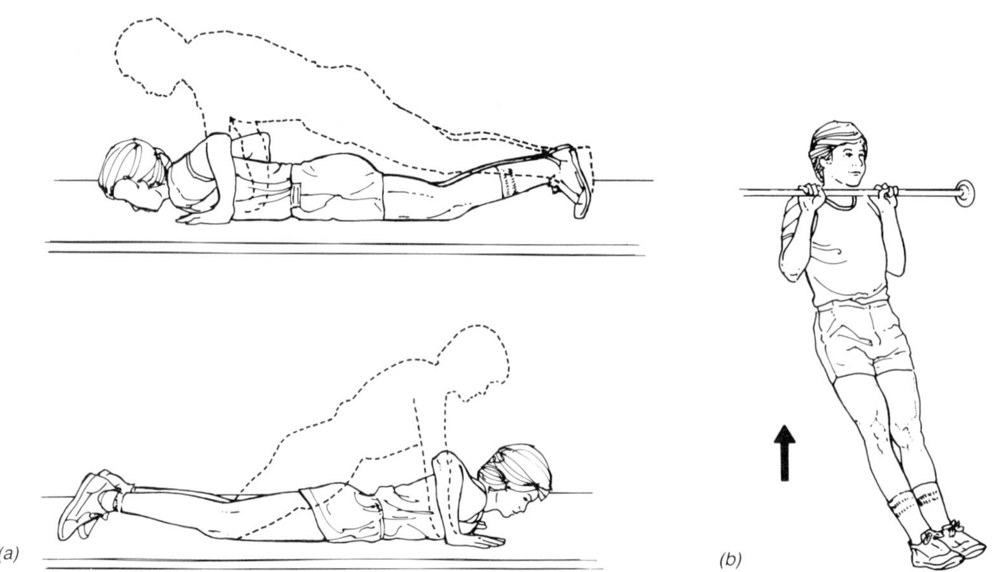

(a)

(b)

Figure 4.4   Measuring dynamic muscular endurance. (a) *Regular push-ups* are done with the subject in a prone position (face downward). The hands should be placed flat on the floor, beside the chest, with the fingers forward. With the body held rigid, the arms are extended completely and then bent again to lower the chest to the floor. This is one push-up, and is repeated as many times as possible without resting in between. *Modified push-ups* are performed in the same way except that the knees, instead of the feet, remain in contact with the floor.

(b) *Pull-ups* are done by jumping to a hanging position on the bar. After hanging for about one second, the subject pulls himself/herself up until the chin comes to the bar and then lets himself/herself down until the elbows are completely straight. This is repeated as many times as possible without rest.

Table 4.4 Dynamic muscular endurance for push-ups, pull-ups, and sit-ups

| | Push-ups | | | | Sit-ups (no./30sec) | |
| | Regular | | Modified | | | |
Percentile	Males (total)	Females (no./30 sec)	Females (total)	Pull-ups Males (total)	Males	Females
90	37	30	40	13	52	40
80	34	26	33	12	48	36
70	31	23	30	11	46	34
60	29	20	27	10	42	30
50	28	16	25	9	40	27
40	26	13	22	8	38	23
30	24	9	18	7	35	22
20	23	6	15	6	32	19
10	20	3	9	4	28	14

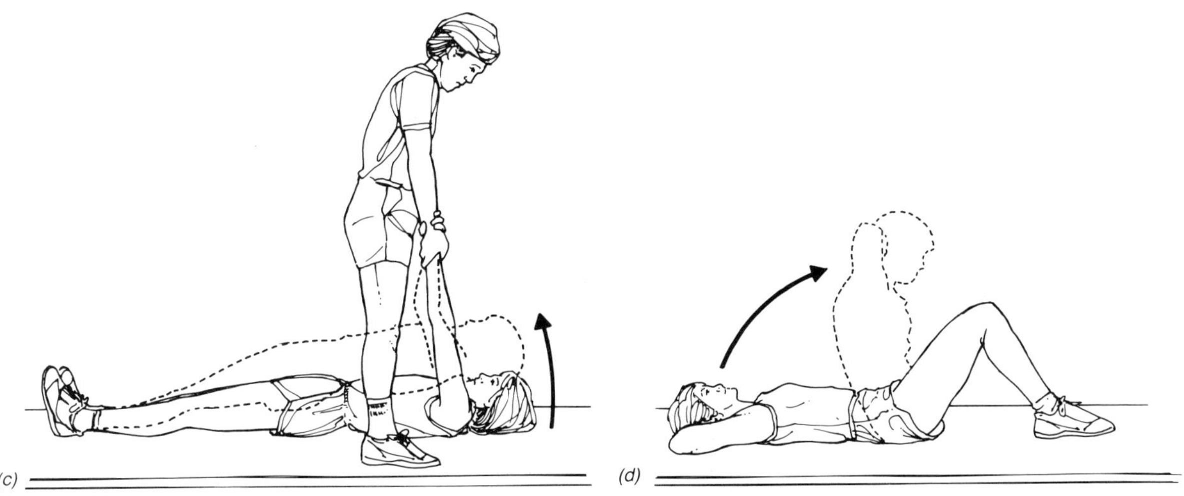

(c) *Modified pull-ups or partner-chins* are done with the performer lying in a supine position (face up) and the partner standing with legs straddling the performer as shown. With partner's hands grasped, the performer bends the elbows until the chest touches the partner's legs. Elbows should be bent at right angles. The arms are then straightened until the performer is again lying on the floor. This is repeated as many times as possible without rest.

(d) *Sit-ups* are done with the legs bent as shown. A partner should hold the subject's feet flat on the floor. The hands are clasped behind the head and the trunk rolled up off the floor, one vertebra at a time, in a curling motion until the chin touches the knees. The performer then returns to the supine position by uncurling slowly. This is repeated as many times as possible without rest.

Muscular power

Muscular power is the amount of work that can be accomplished in a very brief period of time. Both the strength and speed with which you can perform are important for this measurement.

Performance in the shot-put, javelin, or discus is dependent to a considerable extent on the capacity of an individual to generate muscular power. The height you can jump from a crouched position—the vertical jump—is a test of this capacity (Figure 4.5).

Table 4.5 provides some standards for the vertical jump. This measurement is in relative terms by its very nature.

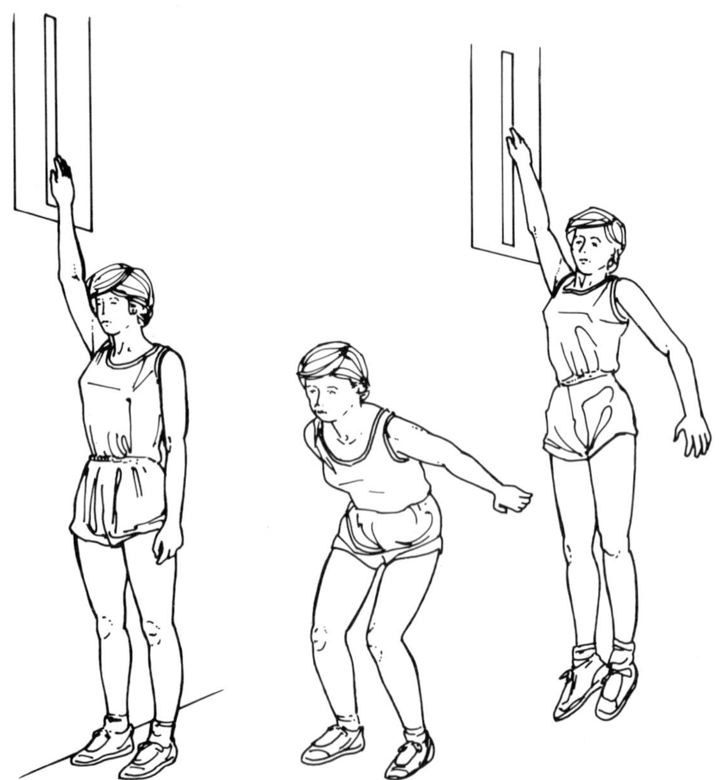

Figure 4.5   Measuring muscular power by doing the vertical jump. The person being tested stands next to the board (or wall) and touches the board as high up as possible while keeping the heels on the floor; this "stretched height" is recorded. The performer then assumes a crouched position and jumps upward and touches the board at the top of the jump as high up as possible. The "jump height" is recorded and the difference between the stretched height and the jump height constitutes the score. Three trials should be made with the maximum height difference being the final score.

Table 4.5 Muscular power of college students doing the vertical jump

	Height difference (inches)	
Percentile	Males	Females
90	25	14
80	24	13
70	23	12
60	19	10
50	16	8
40	13	6
30	9	4
20	8	2
10	2	1

How Flexible Are You?

Basically **flexibility** describes the range of motion around a joint or several joints.

Flexibility: The range of motion around a joint.

Flexibility is important to the performance of many activities; gymnastics and dance require an exceptional degree of flexibility. But even for people who are not involved in those particular pursuits, maintenance of an adequate range of motion in joints is an important aspect of fitness.

Among Americans, flexibility appears to decrease almost continuously from birth to old age. The most obvious example is the loss of flexibility in the hip joint. This is not necessarily a natural consequence of aging, but is probably due to changes in our lifestyles and/or to disabilities we may develop as we get older. If a person has no prohibitive physical problems, general flexibility can be maintained in most people by frequent stretching exercises.

A simple test of hip joint and back flexibility is the sit-and-reach test illustrated in Figure 4.6. Percentile scores for college-age men and women are given in Table 4.6.

Are You a Candidate for Lower Back Pain?

Lower back pain is a common physical complaint. People who have poor flexibility in their hip joints and poor strength in their abdominal muscles are at high risk of experiencing lower back pain. A series of six tests, called Kraus-Weber tests, has been developed to help identify likely candidates for this condition.

The Kraus-Weber tests yield a different type of outcome from the other tests given in this chapter. They are scored on a pass-fail basis, rather than on points within a range that goes from lowest to highest possible achievement. They test for only a low level of fitness, so passing them is not an indication of excellence. Their purpose is simply

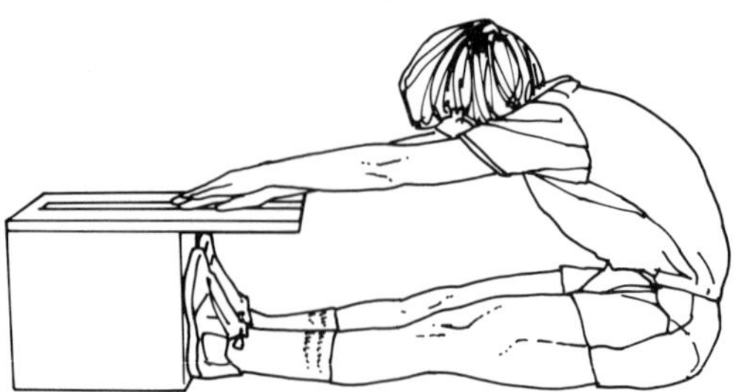

Figure 4.6   Measuring hip flexibility doing the sit-and-reach test. A meter stick is attached to the bench as shown with the numbers increasing away from the subject and the 23 cm mark coinciding with the top edge of the bench, i.e., in line with the bottom of the subject's feet. In the starting position, the performer has knees fully extended and feet flat against the board, shoulder-width apart. The arms are extended, one hand on top of the other, with palms down. The person then bends forward reaching as far as possible and holds this maximum reach for at least one second. The number on the stick closest to the fingertips is the score. Four trials are made and the best score used.

Table 4.6   Joint flexibility of college students doing the sit-and-reach test

| | Reach difference (cm)[a] | |
Percentile	Males	Females
90	40	41
80	37	38
70	35	35
60	33	33
50	30	31
40	28	29
30	25	26
20	21	23
10	15	15

[a]Measured in centimeters reached with the measuring stick extending 23 cm in front of the bench.

to identify those individuals who are at risk of developing lower back pain.

If you want to take the tests, first find a partner to help you. Then proceed as described in the text and as illustrated in Figure 4.7. (Each test is performed once.)

Figure 4.7   Determining whether you are at risk for lower back pain: the Kraus-Weber tests. Instructions are given in the text. If you fail any of these, you are a candidate for lower back pain.

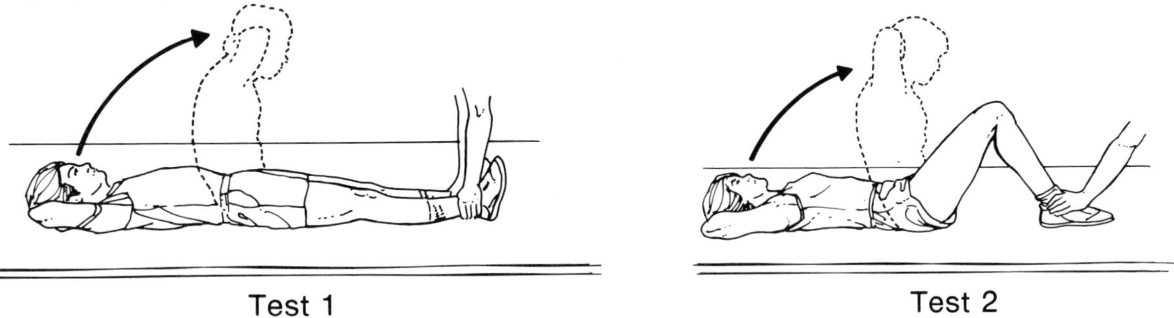

Test 1   Test 2

1. *Straight-leg sit-up*   Lie face up on the floor with hands behind your neck. While your partner holds your feet down, roll up into a sitting position.
2. *Bent-leg sit-up*   Lie face up on the floor with hands behind your neck. With knees bent and bottoms of feet flat on the floor, roll up into a sitting position.

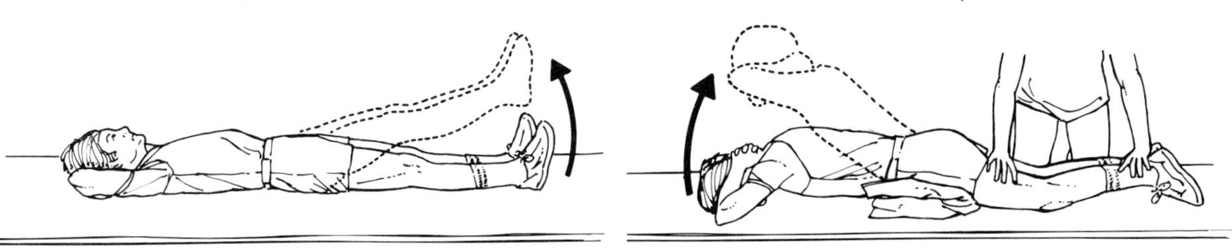

Test 3   Test 4

3. *Forward leg lift*   Lie face up on the floor with hands behind your neck. Keep your knees straight and lift your feet ten inches off the floor, holding the position for ten seconds.
4. *Trunk lift*   Lie face down on the floor with a pillow under your abdomen. With hands behind your neck and feet held down, raise your trunk and hold this position for ten seconds.

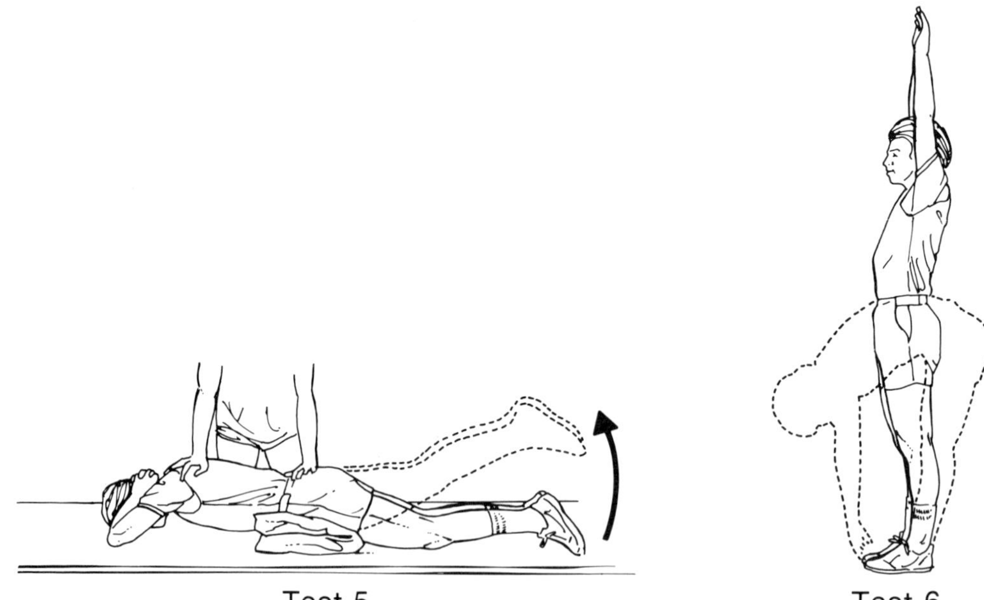

Test 5

Test 6

5. *Backward leg raise* Lie face down on the floor with a pillow under your abdomen and your head cradled on your arms. With back and hips held, lift your legs and hold them off the ground for ten seconds.

6. *Toe touch* Stand erect with legs straight and feet held together. Reach down slowly without straining and touch the floor with your fingertips. Sustain this position for three seconds.

If you fail any of these tests, it would be a good idea for you to begin a program of exercises to improve your strength and/or flexibility up to at least test levels. (Some appropriate exercises are illustrated in Chapter 5.) This can help reduce your risk of developing lower back pain.

Measuring Aerobic Capacity

In Chapter 3, we defined aerobic capacity as being the largest volume of oxygen your body can consume in a minute, which is expressed as maximal oxygen uptake, or $\dot{V}_{O_2}$ max. This is our best estimate of the capacity of your physiological systems to meet the demands of strenuous exercise. It indicates not only the ability of your body cells to generate energy when you are pushing yourself to perform an endurance activity, but it also reflects the capacity of your respiratory and circulatory systems to support that exercise.

For these reasons, aerobic capacity is also commonly referred to as endurance. (Note: This is different from dynamic muscular endurance, which was discussed earlier.) If a test of endurance is a long run (for example, two miles), the score is the time in minutes and seconds required to cover the distance.

Factors That Influence Aerobic Capacity

One factor that has a strong influence on your aerobic capacity or endurance is your *genetic inheritance*; it probably accounts for 60% to 70% of your capacity. That leaves 30% to 40%—still a substantial amount—to be determined by other factors. Let's look at these other determinants.

Aerobic capacity is related to *sex* and *body size*. For young adult men, $\dot{V}_{O_2}$ max averages about 42 milliliters of oxygen per kilogram of body weight per minute (42 ml O_2/kg/min). For young adult women, it averages about 32 ml O_2/kg/min. These sex-related differences exist in part because women have lower blood hemoglobin concentrations and therefore less oxygen-carrying capacity, as was explained in Chapter 3. In addition, in women the size of the heart compared with the total muscle mass is smaller than in men. These factors explain why we give separate standards for men and women, and why $\dot{V}_{O_2}$ max is usually expressed in terms of milliliters of oxygen *per kilogram of body weight* per minute.

These values for maximal oxygen uptake during vigorous exercise stand in sharp contrast to oxygen uptake at rest: at rest, people consume only approximately 3.5 ml O_2/kg/min. Comparing these values, you can see that the average healthy young man has an aerobic capacity of 12 times his resting rate of oxygen consumption, and a woman has approximately 9 times her resting rate.

With such aerobic capacity, a man should be able to sustain a pace of about 8 minutes per mile while running 2 to 3 consecutive miles. A woman should be able to run the same distance at an 11 minute per mile pace.

A simple timed test can be done to evaluate whether a person can achieve these standards. The test involves measuring the distance a person can run in 12 minutes (Balke, 1963; Cooper, 1970). Men should be able to run about 1.6 miles, and women about 1.2 miles in 12 minutes. These are reasonable goals to try to maintain over a lifetime. Table 4.7 shows how college-age men and women were distributed in their performance in this test.

Even if you meet the aerobic capacity standard for your sex today, there is no guarantee that you will maintain it into the future: $\dot{V}_{O_2}$ max is not a fixed value for an individual. Let's look at some of the other factors that influence endurance.

Aerobic activity has a marked effect on aerobic capacity; $\dot{V}_{O_2}$ max increases or is maintained when you do aerobic exercise regularly, but it drifts back down to nonexercise levels during the months after training is discontinued. For example, let's say that you were able to swim a mile in 35 minutes when you were swimming regularly during the summer. You stopped exercising in fall. In winter, you decided to start swimming again; but you found it took you 42 minutes to swim the mile then. This is largely a consequence of loss of aerobic capacity.

Figure 4.8 shows how the aerobic capacities of men of different physical activity levels compare. A graph for women would be similar, although the $\dot{V}_{O_2}$ max values would be lower for each group.

From Figure 4.8 it also appears that *aging* is a factor in the decline of $\dot{V}_{O_2}$ max. However, some physiologists suggest that this loss of capacity need not inevitably occur in concert with the ticking of our biological clocks. They suggest that there may be other possible reasons for this decrease. For one thing, we tend to exercise less vigorously and faithfully as we age than we did when we were younger; the negative effect of this on aerobic capacity was discussed in the paragraph above. We also tend to gain *body fat* with age, and fat acts as "dead weight": people with more fat usually have lower aerobic capacities than people who are leaner. Figure 4.9 shows the relationship

Table 4.7   Running ability of college students for a 12-minute run

| | No. of laps | | | Speed | | Estimated $\dot{V}_{O_2}$ max (ml/kg/ min) |
Percentile	440-yd or 400-m track[a]	0.1-mile track[b]	Distance (miles)	mph	m/min	
Males						
90	6¾	17	1.69	8.4	225	47.2
80	6⅝	16½	1.66	8.3	221	45.8
70	6⅜	16	1.59	8.0	212	44.9
60	6¼	15½	1.56	7.8	208	43.8
50	6	15	1.50	7.5	200	42.4
40	5¾	14½	1.44	7.2	192	41.0
30	5⅝	14	1.41	7.0	188	40.1
20	5⅜	13½	1.34	6.7	179	39.0
10	5¼	13	1.31	6.6	175	37.6
Females						
90	5¼	13	1.31	6.6	175	38.0
80	5	12½	1.25	6.2	167	35.9
70	4⅝	11½	1.16	5.8	154	34.4
60	4⅜	11	1.09	5.5	146	32.8
50	4¼	10½	1.06	5.3	142	31.8
40	4	10	1.00	5.0	133	30.5
30	3¾	9½	0.94	4.7	125	29.2
20	3⅝	9	0.91	4.5	121	27.6
10	3¼	8	0.81	4.0	108	25.4

[a]Total number of laps run in 12 minutes on either a 440-yard or a 400-meter track.
[b]Total number of laps run in 12 minutes on a 0.1-mile track.

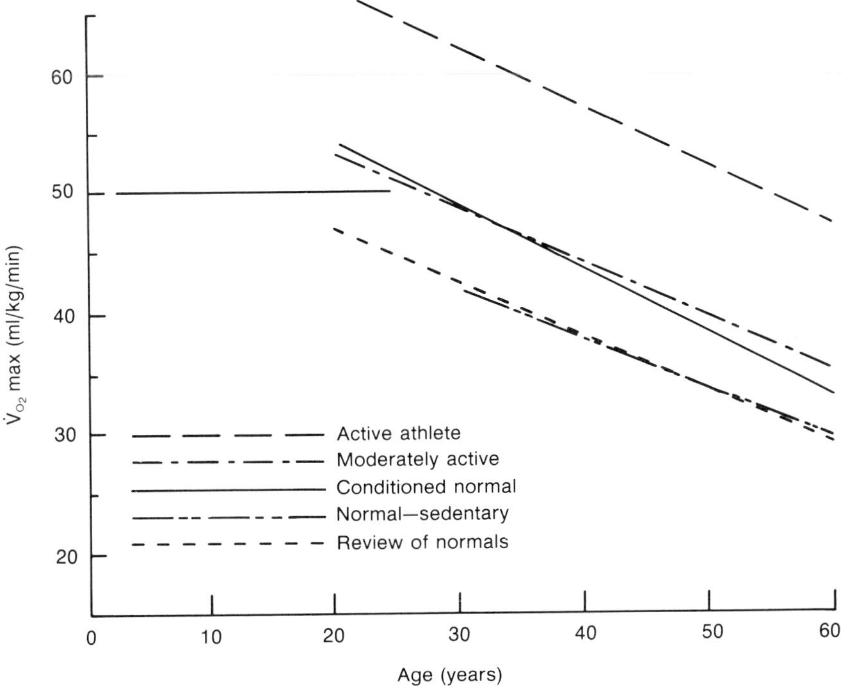

Figure 4.8 The relationship between maximal oxygen uptake ($\dot{V}_{O_2}$ max) and age for men at different physical activity levels. "Review of Normals" refers to a summary of studies of nonathletes.

between age, body fatness, and aerobic capacity.

Perhaps the most persuasive reason for not accepting the idea that aging *inevitably* produces decreasing aerobic capacity comes from a study, as yet unpublished, that involves former college athletes who have continued to exercise aerobically. The study shows that these former athletes, who now are over 50 years of age, have *not* lost significant aerobic capacity over the decades. Such research suggests that loss of endurance may have more to do with muscle disuse and increase in body weight than with aging itself.

Another factor that produces a lower $\dot{V}_{O_2}$ max is *smoking* (Montoye et al., 1980). This occurs for the following reasons:

1. Smoking decreases the amount of air that can be taken into the lungs.
2. Smoking causes changes in the lungs which inhibit exchange of gases between lungs and blood.
3. Carbon monoxide in smoke binds to hemoglobin and therefore decreases the amount of oxygen the blood can carry.
4. Hormones produced by the body in response to smoking may cause a restriction of blood flow to muscle, thereby limiting oxygen utilization.

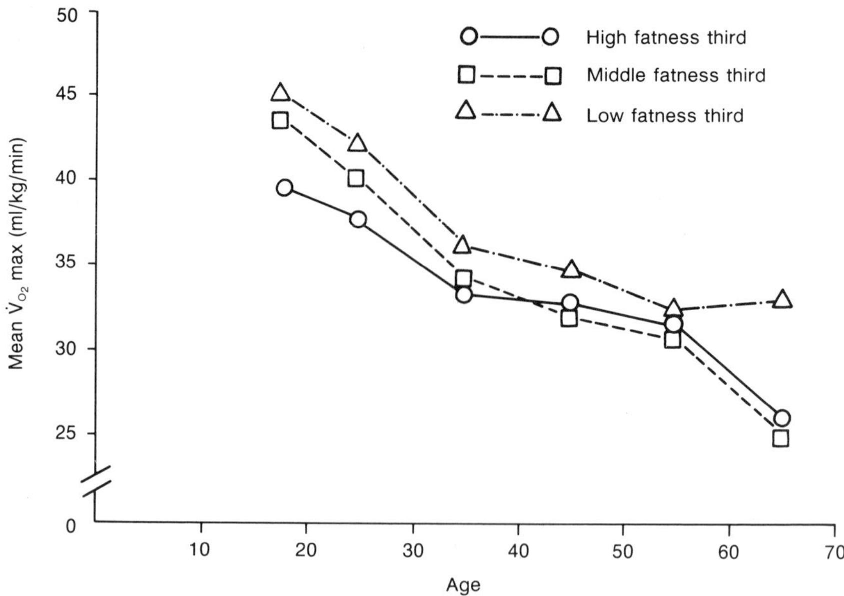

Figure 4.9 The relationship between maximal oxygen uptake ($\dot{V}_{O_2}$ max) and body fatness in males.

Estimating resting oxygen requirement

From the fact that a person uses approximately 3.5 O_2/kg/min at rest, you can estimate the amount of oxygen you use at rest by multiplying the above value by your weight in kilograms.

We will use Maria as an example. She weighs 132 pounds, which is equal to 60 kg, since there are 2.2 lb/kg. Now the problem looks like this:

$$O_2 \text{ use at rest} = 3.5 \text{ ml } O_2 \text{ kg/ml} \times 60 \text{ kg} = 210 \text{ ml } O_2/\text{min}$$

To convert from milliliters to liters, you must divide by 1,000 since there are 1,000 milliliters in a liter. Therefore:

$$210 \text{ ml } O_2/\text{min} \div 1,000 = 0.21 \text{ liters } O_2/\text{min}$$

Resting metabolic rate (RMR): The amount of oxygen and/or the energy per unit of time needed to keep a person alive.

This is the amount of oxygen Maria uses just for keeping herself alive; it represents her **resting metabolic rate (RMR)**. It does not include the amount that she uses for physical activity or for metabolizing food for several hours after a meal. We discuss resting oxygen consumption because, as the reader will see, the energy cost of activities are generally expressed in multiples of the resting oxygen consumption.

Use the first formula of Self-check 4.1 to calculate the volume of oxygen you use at rest.

Self-check 4.1   Estimating resting metabolic rate (RMR)

1. Write your body weight in kilograms in the first blank.

    O_2 use at rest = 3.5 ml O_2/kg/min × _______ kg = _______ ml O_2/min

    _______ ml O_2/min ÷ 1000 = _______ liters O_2/min

2. RMR per minute = _______ liters O_2/min × 5 kcal/liter = _______ kcal/min

    RMR per hour = _______ kcal/min × 60 min/hr = _______ kcal/hr

    RMR per day = _______ kcal/hr × 24 hr/day = _______ kcal/day

Energy expenditure and oxygen consumption

There is a direct relationship between the total amount of oxygen consumed and the energy expended. For every liter of oxygen you take up, you use 5 kcalories. Therefore if you know how much oxygen you have used, you can calculate the amount of energy you expended. Let's calculate how much energy Maria uses at rest: 0.21 liters/min × 5 kcal/liter = 1.05 kcal/min.

Of course, you can extend this calculation to determine what the kcaloric expenditure would be at rest for an hour or a whole day. In Maria's case, for 1 hour it would be: 1.05 kcal/min × 60 min/hr = 63 kcal/hr. For 1 day it would be 63 kcal/hr × 24 hr/day = 1,512 kcal/day.

These values are alternative ways of expressing the resting metabolic rate. The lower part of Self-check 4.1 provides the space for determining your resting metabolic rate.

Calculating energy expenditure using METS

As you know from Chapter 3, during physical activity the body's demand for oxygen increases. Physiologists have found it convenient to express this increased demand in terms of multiples of the amount of oxygen consumed at rest, which they refer to as **METS**. One MET equals 3.5 ml O_2/kg/min, or in other words, normal oxygen consumption at rest.

METS: Multiples of the amount of oxygen and/or energy used at rest.

Exercise physiologists have tested many people doing various activities, and have established approximate MET values for different types of work and play. MET values therefore provide a convenient means of comparing the intensity of various activities.

For example, the intensity of walking is 3.5 METS; that is, you use 3.5 times as much oxygen (and therefore energy) for walking as for resting. Jogging (12 min/mile) has an intensity of 8.5 METS; it costs you eight and one-half times as much energy as resting does.

Tables 4.8 and 4.9 list the intensities of various activities in METS. Once you know the MET value of an activity, you can find out how much energy you would expend per minute by multiplying it by your RMR, which you calculated in Self-check 4.1:

$$\text{kcal/min} = \underline{\hspace{2em}} \text{ METS} \times \text{RMR in kcal/min} = \underline{\hspace{2em}} \text{ kcal/min}$$

Maria, whose RMR is 1.05 kcal/min, could expect to expend while jogging:

$$8.5 \text{ METS} \times 1.05 \text{ kcal/min} = 8.9 \text{ kcal/min}$$

Table 4.8   MET values for various school and job activities

Type of activity	Intensity (METS)
Sitting: light or moderate work	
Sitting at desk, writing, calculating	1.5
Driving a car	1.5
Using hand tools, light assembly work	1.8
Driving a truck (no loading, unloading)	1.8
Working heavy levers, dredge	2.0
Riding mower	2.5
Driving heavy truck or trailer rig (incl. getting on and off frequently and doing some arm work)	3.0
Standing: moderate work	
Standing quietly, working at own pace; laboratory work, bartending, clerking	2.5
Using hand tools (e.g., gas station operator)	2.7
Scrubbing, waxing, polishing	2.7
Assembling or repairing heavy machine parts, e.g., farm machinery, plumbing	3.0
Light welding	3.0
Stocking shelves: packing/unpacking small or medium-sized objects; most jobs in fast food restaurants	3.0
Sanding floors with a power sander	3.0
Assembling light or medium machine parts at rate of 500 times per day or more	3.5
Assembling and lifting (at approx. 5-min intervals) parts up to 45 lb	3.5
Assembling and lifting (at approx. 5-min intervals) parts over 45 lb	4.0
Cranking up dollies, hitching trailers, operating large levers	3.5
Pulling on wires, twisting cables	3.5
Masonry, painting, paperhanging	4.0
Walking: moderate work	
Walking	3.5
Carrying trays, dishes, etc.	4.2
Walking during gas station mechanic work	4.5

(Continued)

Table 4.8 Continued

Type of activity	Intensity (METS)
Standing and/or walking: heavy arm work	
Lifting and carrying objects:	
20–44 lb object	4.5
45–64 lb object	6.0
65–84 lb object	7.5
85–100 lb object	8.5
Heavy tools:	
Pneumatic tools (jackhammers, drills, spades, tampers)	6.0
Shovel, pick, tunnel bar	8.0
Moving, pushing heavy objects (75 lb or more)	8.0
Carpentry	6.0
General heavy industrial work	5.0
Other:	
Laying railroad track	7.0
Cutting trees, chopping wood:	
Power saw	3.0
Hand saw or axe	5.5

Table 4.9 MET values for various active leisure and discretionary time activities

Type of activity	Intensity (METS)
Archery (not hunting)	3.5
Backpacking	7.0
Badminton	7.0
Basketball, competitive	10.0
Basketball, recreational	6.0
Bicycling, level, 14 MPH	2.5
Bicycling, level, 24 MPH	5.0
Bicycling, competitively	12.0
Bowling	3.0
Calisthenics, home exercise	4.5
Canoeing or rowing leisurely	3.5
Canoeing on a camping trip	4.0
Canoeing or rowing competitively	12.0
Cross-country hiking	6.0
Dancing, aerobic	6.0
Dancing, ballroom	3.0
Dancing, square, folk, or modern	6.0
Fencing	5.5
Fishing from boat or on ice	2.0
Fishing from river bank	3.5
Fishing in stream with wading boots	6.0

(Continued)

Table 4.9 Continued

Type of activity	Intensity (METS)
Football, touch or tackle	6.0
Gardening, spading and digging	5.0
Gardening, weeding and cultivating	4.5
Golf, using power cart, 9 holes/hr	3.0
Golf, pull cart for clubs, 9 holes/1½ hr	5.0
Golf, carrying clubs, 9 holes/1½ hr	5.0
Gymnastics	5.5
Handball	8.0
Hockey	8.0
Horseback riding	3.5
Horseshoe pitching	3.0
Hunting, including bow hunting	5.0
Jogging or running, level (12-min/mile)	8.5
Jogging or running, 2.5% grade (12-min/mile)	10.5
Jogging or running, level (8-min/mile)	12.5
Jogging or running, 2.5% grade (8-min/mile)	15.0
Mountain climbing	8.0
Mowing lawn, riding mower	2.5
Mowing lawn, walking behind power mower	4.0
Mowing lawn, walking behind hand mower	5.5
Paddleball	8.0
Power boating	2.0
Racketball	8.0
Raking lawn	4.0
Sailing	3.0
Scuba diving	7.0
Skating, ice or roller	7.0
Skiing, downhill; first lift until skis off	4.0
Skiing, cross-country	8.0
Sledding or tobogganing	7.0
Snorkeling	5.0
Snow shoveling	6.0
Soccer	8.0
Softball	5.0
Squash	8.0
Swimming, recreational	6.0
Swimming, competitive	8.0–12.0
Table tennis	4.0
Tennis, doubles	6.0
Tennis, singles	7.0
Volleyball	4.0
Walking	3.5
Water-skiing	6.0
Weight lifting, health club	4.5
Wrestling or judo	8.0

Measuring anaerobic capacity

Unfortunately, for those interested in information regarding testing and enhancing anaerobic capacity, we don't have much to offer. Tests of anaerobic capacity involve such precise measurement that they are difficult to do in the typical athletic department or fitness center. It is not known to what extent anaerobic capacity is an inherited trait, or to what extent training might be able to influence it.

MET values are also very useful for assessing your overall activity level. This section will explain how to use the information in Table 4.8, Table 4.9, and in Self-check 4.1 for estimating your overall activity level. The form on which to do your assessment is found in Self-check 4.2. Figure 4.10 provides an example of one student's activity self-assessment using this form.

Activity Level and Energy Expenditure

The objective is to account for all 168 hours of a typical week by determining how many hours are usually spent in each type of activity. Notice that there are several different categories of activity that need to be filled in: eating meals, sleeping, student and job activities, active leisure activities, and quiet leisure.

Here are the steps for filling out the form:

1. *Eating*   Estimate the total number of hours per week you spend eating. Enter this number in the second column.

2. *Sleeping*   Estimate the number of hours you spend per week sleeping. Enter this number in the second column.

3. *Student and job activities*   Add up the number of hours you are seated in class each week. Enter the number in the second column. If you have any laboratory classes in which you stand, list "Labs" on the next line; then enter the MET value for laboratory work (2.5 METS, as shown in Table 4.8) in the first column on the left; then enter the hours per week you are in the lab. If you have a job, find the closest description of what you do in Table 4.8; then, just as was described for lab work, enter METS and time.

4. *Active leisure and discretionary time activities*   Next, estimate the number of hours you spend per week in the activities shown in Table 4.9. List them in the same way as you did your student and job activities in the previous section. If an activity that you did is not listed in Table 4.9, use the value of an activity that seems similar in the amount of effort involved.

5. *Quiet leisure*   Total the number of hours from all sections. The sum is likely to fall short of the 168 hours in the week, because you probably spent some quiet leisure time that you haven't yet accounted for. To calculate how much time was involved in quiet

leisure, subtract the sum you just calculated from 168; enter this figure in the hours/week column across from quiet leisure.

6. *Intensity × time*   Then multiply each intensity value (METS) by the time in hours per week and record in the third column.

7. *Average intensity (METS) per hour*   Now total the far right column. Divide the sum by 168 (hours in the week). Your answer indicates what your overall intensity is per hour, averaged for the whole week. Table 4.10 gives the percentile distribution for college-age men and women.

8. *Average daily energy expenditure*   Multiply your average intensity per hour by 24 (hours in a day) and by the number of kcalories you use per hour at rest (from Self-check 4.1). Your

Self-check 4.2   Estimating overall activity level and energy expenditure

Activity	Intensity (METS)	Time (hrs/week)	Intensity × time
Eating	1.8		
Sleeping	1.0		
Student, job activities: sitting	1.5		
Active leisure activities:			
Quiet leisure	1.8		
	TOTAL	168	

Your average METS per hour equals the total METS for the week (see the total in column three) divided by 168 (the number of hours per week):

_______ METS/week ÷ 168 hrs/week = _______ METS/hr

Your average energy (kcal) expenditure for a day equals your RMR in kcal/hr (see Self-check 4.1) × 24 hrs per day × your average METS per hour:

_______ kcal/hr × 24 hrs/day × _______ METS/hr = _______ kcal/day

answer indicates what your approximate daily kcalorie expenditure is, averaged for the whole week.

$$\text{Daily energy use} = \text{average METS/hr} \times 24 \times \text{RMR/hr}$$

For Alan, the student whose activity assessment appears in Figure 4.10, the average METS/hr value was 1.73. In an earlier assessment he learned that his resting metabolic rate was 66 kcalories per hour. Therefore his average daily energy use would be:

$$\text{Daily energy use} = 1.73 \times 24 \text{ hr} \times 66 \text{ kcal/hr} = 2740 \text{ kcal}$$

Figure 4.10   An example of a filled-in form of Self-check 4.2, showing how Alan evaluated his actual weekly activity.

Activity	Intensity (METS)	Time (hrs/week)	Intensity × time
Eating	1.8	4.7	8.5
Sleeping	1.0	51.0	51.0
Student, job activities: sitting (class + studying)	1.5	31.0	46.5
labs	2.5	6.0	15.0
janitor job	2.7	15.0	40.5
Active leisure activities: bicycling, leisurely	4.0	3.2	12.8
table tennis	4.0	.7	2.8
volleyball	4.0	1.5	6.0
walking	3.5	5.0	17.5
Quiet leisure	1.8	49.9	89.8
	TOTAL	168	290.4

Your average METS per hour equals the total METS for the week (see the total in column three) divided by 168 (the number of hours per week):

290.4 METS/week ÷ 168 hrs/week = 1.73 METS/hr

Your average energy (kcal) expenditure for a day equals your RMR in kcal/hr (see Self-check 4.1) × 24 hrs per day × your average METS per hour:

66 kcal/hr × 24 hrs/day × 1.73 METS/hr = 2740 kcal/day

Table 4.10 Average activity intensity of college students

Percentile	Intensity (METS/hr)[a]	
	Males	Females
90 (most active)	2.18	2.06
80	2.04	1.95
70	1.95	1.89
60	1.89	1.84
50	1.84	1.80
40	1.80	1.76
30	1.77	1.72
20	1.74	1.67
10	1.65	1.59
Number of subjects	59	123

[a]The rate is the average value over a 1-week period.

Such energy expenditure information is especially useful if you want to gain or lose weight. Knowing your energy expenditure is the same as knowing what kcalorie intake is required to keep your body weight stable. If you want to gain or lose weight, energy expenditure can be adjusted down or up. This will be discussed in the body weight chapter.

What Ratings Should You Try to Achieve?

The assessments in this chapter have given you some methods for discovering how you rate in strength, flexibility, aerobic capacity, overall activity, and energy expenditure. For most of these measures, we have provided tables of distribution that enable you to compare your own performance to that of many people of your age and sex.

But what level of fitness should you try to achieve? Should you strive for the 95th percentile or above? Or is it reasonable to be satisfied with the 50th? Here are some thoughts to keep in mind regarding use of the percentile rankings. First of all, we need to acknowledge again that each of us has physiological limits as to what maximal levels of fitness we can achieve. Our genetic inheritance affects each aspect of performance, and some people have additional limits imposed by illness or injury; therefore most of us would be unable to perform at the 95th percentile even if we undertook the ultimate training program. There are no uniform, standard percentiles that represent adequate fitness for everybody, because we vary in our physiological ability to attain them.

In that light, you can see that a person at the 50th percentile who exercises regularly might actually be in better condition *relative to his potential* than somebody else who is at the 60th percentile but is not physically active. The person at the 60th percentile should not feel smug about his higher ranking; he or she might be able to do more to improve his fitness than his cohort at the 50th.

Therefore, rather than attaching a great deal of importance to a specific percentile for goal-setting purposes, use the figures to give yourself a general idea of your level of functioning. For goal setting, physiologists usually encourage people to think in terms of the following:

- Doing types of exercise that can produce improvement in function
- Exercising often enough and long enough to produce improvement in function
- Exercising hard enough to bring about improvement in function, but not so hard as to result in injury

Ways to set up such a program are discussed in Chapter 5.

After you have designed and used your individualized program for a time, you can reassess what gains you have made in functional capacity by repeating the tests in this chapter. If you reach a higher percentile on the second assessment than on the first, you know that your program is working. Being able to make such comparisons is another value of using these tests.

Now let's move on to Chapter 5 to find out about how to set up your own individualized exercise program.

Exercise Programs for Fitness

5

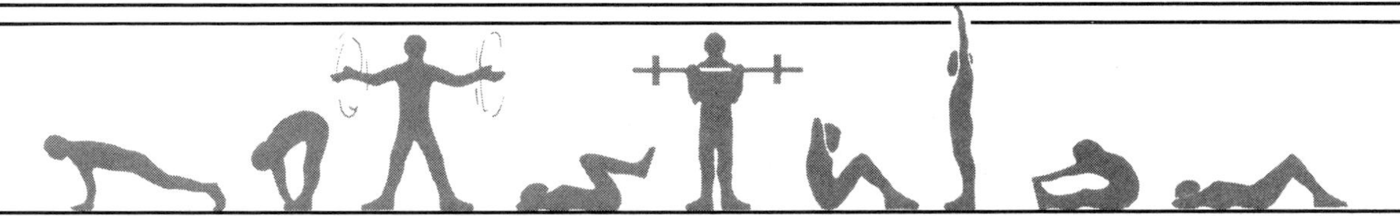

Outline

We have acknowledged in previous chapters that over the centuries the day-to-day activities of people—whether students or employees or householders or all three—have generally come to require less and less physical activity. Therefore, today it is our leisure time that offers us the opportunity to increase physical activity and improve fitness.

But on what basis should people choose their activities?

Most often, people choose their activities based on how well they enjoy participation. Perhaps you like a certain form of exercise because you're good at it, or because you have friends who are also interested in that activity, or because it makes you feel better physically or mentally. That's all to the good: if you like an activity, chances are that you will do it long enough, hard enough, and often enough to reap the benefits it can provide. But liking a particular type of exercise is not the only important criterion for choosing it.

Consider both the benefits and limitations of various types of exercise. For example, weight lifting increases strength, but not flexibility or aerobic capacity to any great degree; running increases aerobic capacity but not upper body strength or flexibility; and gymnastics increase flexibility and overall strength but not necessarily aerobic capacity. Therefore a given type of exercise can provide specific benefits with very little carryover.

The best program, then, involves several different types of exercise that offer improvement in all aspects of fitness—*strength, flexibility*, and *aerobic capacity (endurance)*. A good program design has to consider your fitness starting point, so that you do not overtax yourself and get discouraged at the outset. This is particularly important for people who have not found an activity that they enjoy, and may be looking for a convenient excuse to quit the program right at the start.

Therefore, we will focus here on the types of exercise that can be enjoyed by people over their entire lifetimes. We do not put major emphasis on the use of very sophisticated and expensive exercise machines—although many of them may be useful, they are inaccessible to many people over the long term.

There's one more important qualification about this information we are about to present, and that is that these recommendations are only for normally healthy people. If you have a chronic illness or physical disability, you should have the approval of your health care provider and the help of an exercise specialist in tailoring an activity program to your unique needs and abilities.

Now let's look at the recommended features of an exercise program, and then address the problem of how to keep yourself involved in activity.

Go for Strength, Flexibility, and Endurance

First, there are some generalizations that apply to all of the recommendations.

1. *Train, don't strain.* This axiom indicates that when you design an exercise program for yourself, you should start at a level that pushes your performance a bit, but not far enough to cause injury or even acute discomfort. The key is to make your first session slow and easy, and progress gradually in subsequent workouts. Talk to your jogging partner, if that happens to be your type of activity, and when talking becomes difficult you are going too fast. During an exercise session, periodically check how the effort is affecting your body (that means monitoring your heart rate, which will be described shortly), and take it easier when your body tells you to.

2. *Don't hold your breath.* Although this expression is used often in a figurative sense, here we mean it literally. Allow yourself to

breathe normally during exercise. As your exercise intensity increases, your breathing will automatically increase in both rate and depth; this will feel necessary and right to you, and it is. On the other hand, sometimes you may want to hold your breath and strain momentarily during calisthenic or weight training exercises. Try not to do this, because it adds to your sense of physical stress and unduly increases your blood pressure. Neither response is desirable so *breathe normally.*

Increasing your strength

Strength exercises are specific to the muscles they stress.

Here are some suggestions for achieving improvements in strength of various muscle groups.

Neck exercises Neck muscles can be strengthened by doing the resistance exercises shown in Figure 5.1. A strength and endurance *reserve* for neck muscles, especially the neck extensor muscles which are constantly active in our awake and upright posture, is very important. The simple exercises of Figure 5.1 accomplish this goal and also tax the muscles through a wide range of motion which is desirable. Do 8 to 15 repetitions of each.

Arm and upper body exercises We offer two methods—one set of exercises requires little equipment, and the other is done with weights.

The first option involves calisthenics that can be done with a stationary horizontal bar as the only special equipment. Figure 4.4 in the previous chapter illustrates how to do push-ups and pull-ups. For push-ups, many men work toward a goal of 10 to 15 done slowly; women often work toward 7 to 10 regular push-ups done slowly, or 15 to 20 of the modified variety. For pull-ups, strive toward 7 to 10, slowly done; as explained in Chapter 4. Women may do what is called "partner chins" where part of the body weight is supported by the floor.

The second option involves weight training. There are three basic methods of weight training called isotonic, isometric, and isokinetic. Recall that *isotonic* contractions (see Chapter 3) are those in which muscles undergo shortening in contraction, and *isometric* contractions are those in which there is no change in muscle length during contractions. Exercise regimens invoking such muscle responses are identified as isotonic and isometric methods, respectively.

Isokinetic weight training is a special form of the isotonic method. The word isokinetic means the "same motion" or "equal motion." This is interpreted to mean equal rate of motion or equal speed. In **isokinetic contractions**, the rate of muscle shortening is controlled. Special machines are manufactured for isokinetic training that involve some type of hydraulic system or cams and clutches to adjust resistance to muscle tension, to achieve constant speed of shortening.

Isokinetic contraction: A contraction in which the rate of shortening of muscle is controlled by adjustments in the weight being moved.

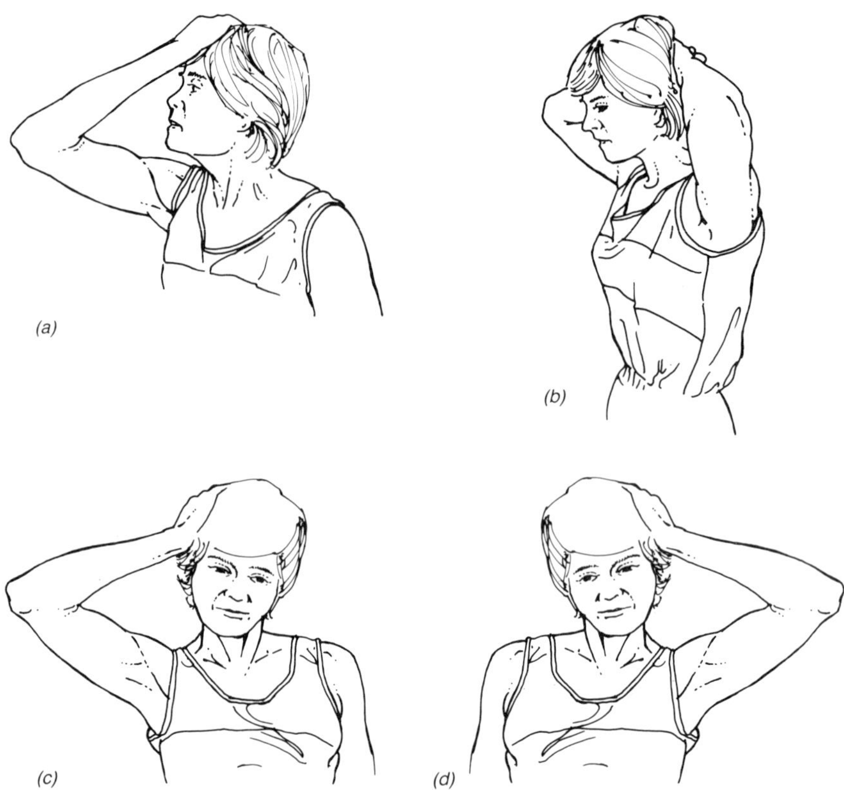

Figure 5.1 Strength exercises for the neck. You can increase the strength of your neck muscles by resisting movements of your head with your hand. Eight to 15 repetitions of each exercise are recommended. (a) Resist flexion movement. From extended head position, attempt to bring chin to chest against resistance. (b) Resist extension movement. From flexed head position, attempt to extend head against resistance. (c) Right lateral flexion. From leftward flexed head position, move right against resistance. (d) Left lateral flexion. From rightward flexed head position, move left against resistance.

While a case can be made for all three types of training methods depending on goals, we will limit our discussion to the more conventional isotonic muscle training method. To use this option, you need dumbbells, barbells, or exercise machines with adjustable resistance. Start with a weight load that allows you to do 8 to 10 repetitions; on subsequent days, gradually increase the number of repetitions you do until you reach 15. At that point, add the next increment of weight (an additional 5 pounds), and do 8 to 10 repetitions with this weight. Gradually increase repetitions to a maximum of 15 in the following sessions. This is an application of the **overload principle**. With 8 to 15 repetitions, contributions are made both to muscle strength and endurance. With more weight and fewer repetitions, the emphasis is on strength; with more repetitions and less weight, the emphasis is on

Overload principle: Adding weight to dumbbell or barbell as an exercise repetition maximum is attained.

sustaining muscular effort, identified as **muscle endurance**.

There are many variations of upper-body exercises. Figure 5.2 illustrates four that provide activity for all of those major muscle groups.

When can you stop adding weights and simply maintain your program? Fitness experts suggest that when you can slowly do 7 to 10 pull-ups you are ready for maintenance. Success in such a test indicates you have adequate strength and endurance to control and project your body weight with your upper body musculature. Of course, some people may wish to further increase the weight they're lifting, either to see what their upper limit of strength might be, or for body-building purposes; such goals go beyond what exercise physiologists think is important for general fitness.

Muscle endurance: Ability of select muscle groups to repeat and/or sustain contractions.

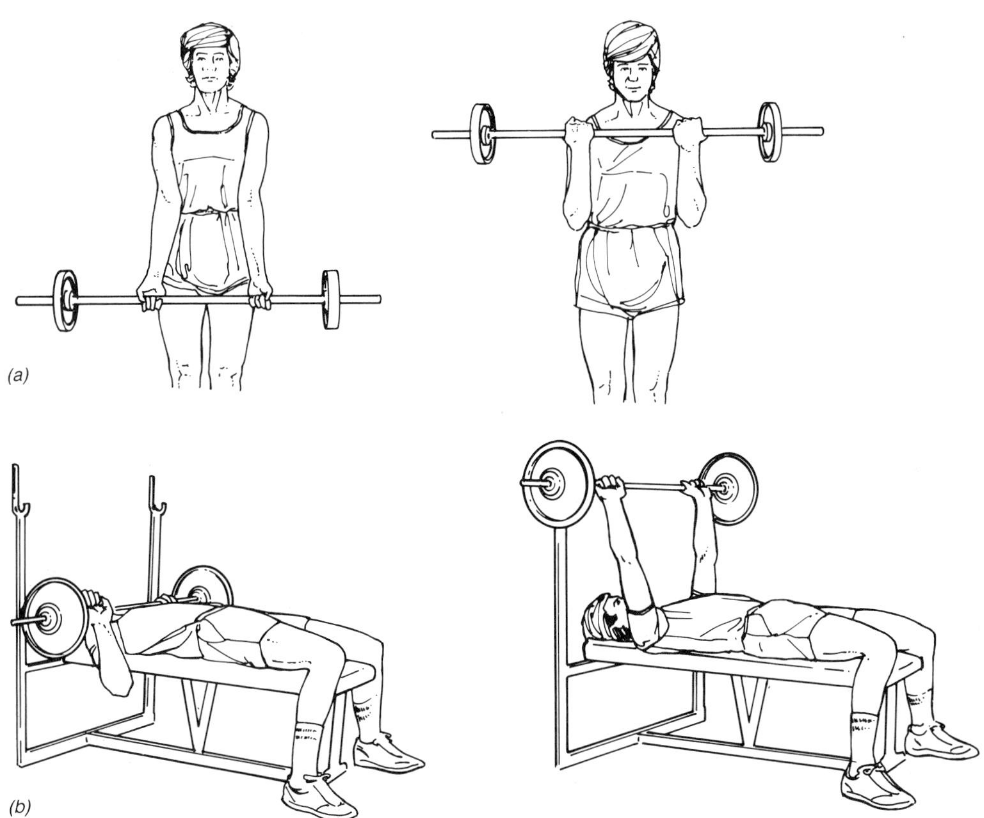

Figure 5.2 Strength exercises (done with weights) for the arms and upper body. Both strength and muscular endurance can be increased with 8 to 15 repetitions.

(a) Arm curl. With feet apart at shoulder width, hold bar at thighs. Bring bar up to shoulders, keeping back straight, then return bar to thighs.

(b) Bench press. Lie face-up on bench with feet on floor, support the bar with hands at chest, then push the bar from chest to extended arm position. Return the bar to chest.

(Continued next page)

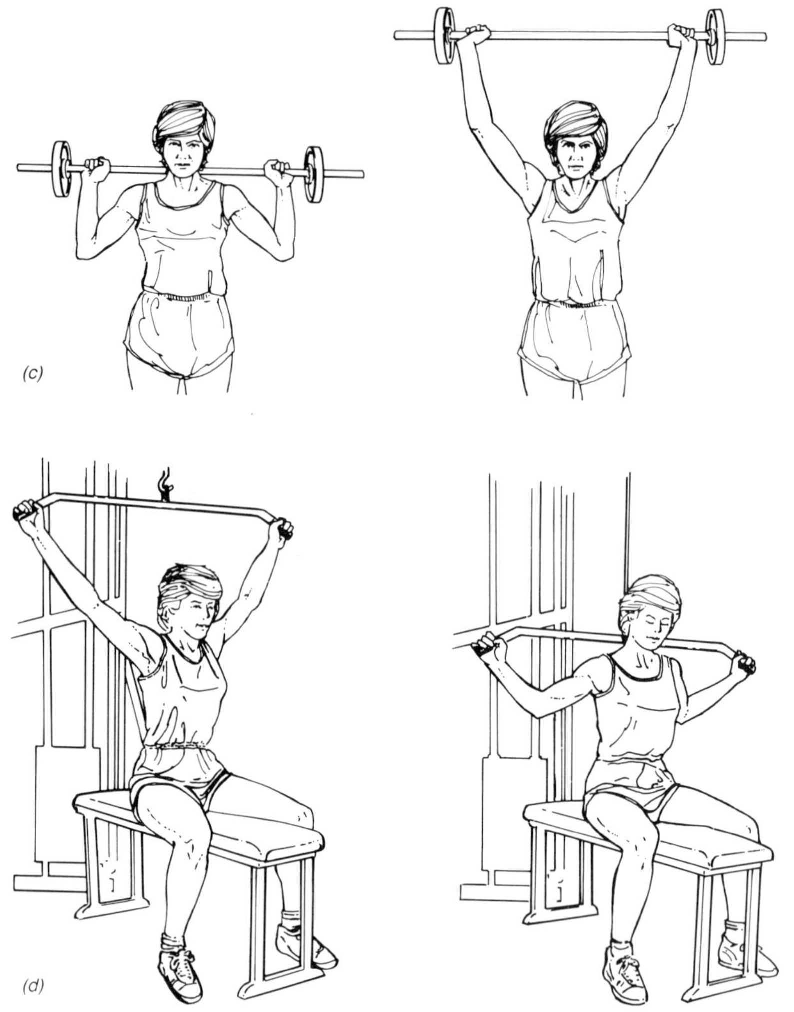

Figure 5.2 (Continued)

(c) Military press. Stand and hold bar on shoulders behind head, extend arms overhead, and return to initial position. The exercise may also be done from a starting position at chest.

(d) Pull-down. This exercise requires the use of Universal Gym equipment. Sit or kneel below bar, with arms extended to grip bar. Pull down against weights and touch the bar to back of neck before returning to initial position.

Abdominal exercises   Sit-ups (Figure 4.4) and pelvic curls (Figure 5.3) strengthen abdominal muscles. During sit-ups, muscles pull from attachments on the pelvis, drawing up the upper portion of the trunk. During pelvic curls, the opposite occurs as abdominal muscles pull from attachments on the ribcage, rotating the pelvis to the chest. In both exercises, lower-back muscles are beneficially stretched as well.

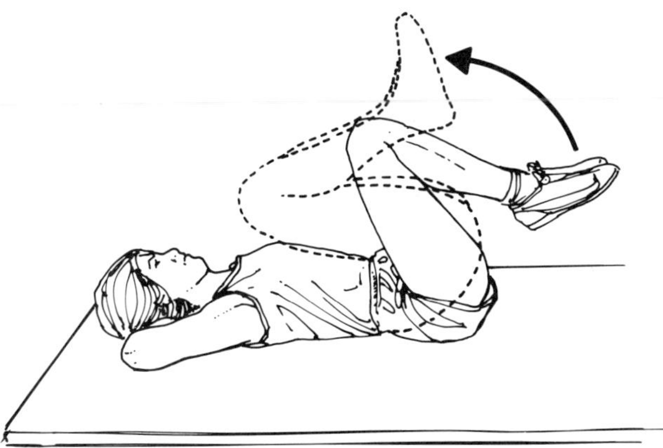

Figure 5.3   Strength exercise for abdominal muscles. Like sit-ups (illustrated in Figure 4.4), pelvic curls strengthen the abdominal muscles. Lie supine, with hands behind head, and flex at hips and knees. Roll pelvis upward, bringing knees toward chin. Return to initial position and rest briefly between repetitions. Ten to 15 repetitions are recommended.

Leg exercises   Many people do not need to seek out special strengthening exercises for their legs because they condition their legs for relative strength while they do their aerobic activities. Distance walkers, runners, bicyclists, skiers, and others develop leg strength and endurance by moving against the resistance of their body weight. Nevertheless, some of these people would benefit from these exercises during the off-season (skiers, for example).

However, such sports as swimming and canoeing, although they have great aerobic benefit, do not substantially increase leg strength. Therefore, a person whose main form of exercise is swimming or canoeing is likely to benefit from leg exercises.

Squats and toe raises (Figure 5.4) will increase leg strength. Progress from 8 to 15 repetitions of each exercise to increase both strength and muscular endurance.

It is not a good idea to work your muscles to the limits of their endurance day after day; it is better to stress them on alternate days to give them a chance to rest in between. If you want to do strength exercises every day, you could do upper body exercises one day and lower body exercises the next.

Increasing your flexibility

Flexibility can be increased by bending and stretching. The joint most in need of flexibility exercise, because of its association with the common problem of lower back pain, is the hip joint.

Figure 5.5 shows exercises that are used to increase the flexibility of the hip joint and to stretch muscles of the legs and back. Do not bounce while doing them; when you bounce, your muscles react by shortening in contraction instead of lengthening in a relaxed state. Therefore

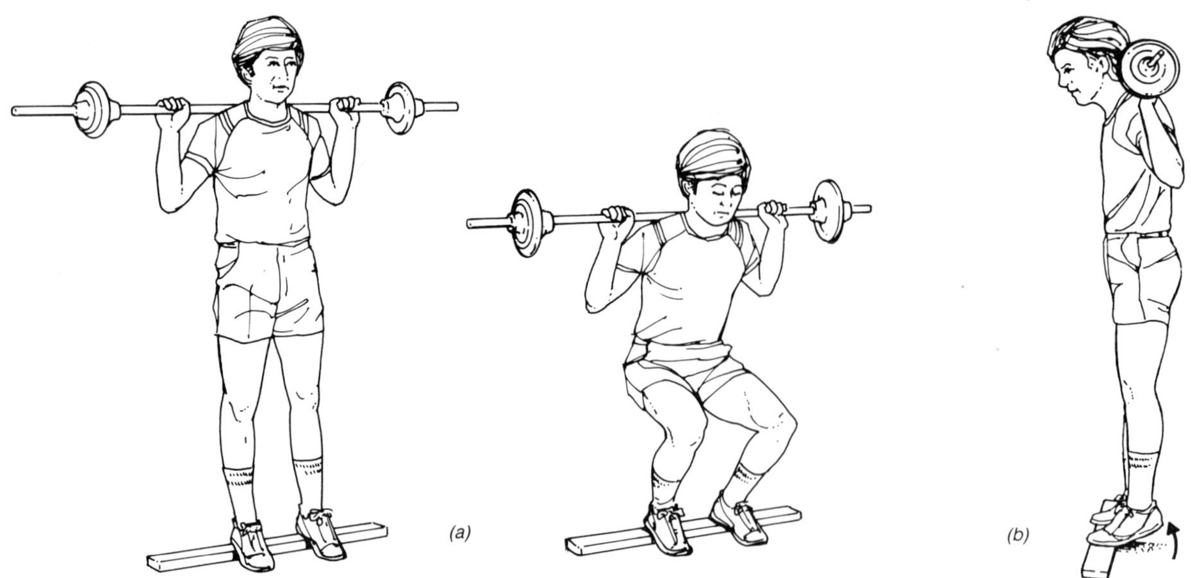

Figure 5.4 Strength exercises for the legs. It is expecially important to begin these exercises with light weights to avoid back injury. (a) Squat. Stand erect, and place the barbell on the shoulders behind the neck. Keeping the back straight, lower the weight by flexing the knees to a 90° angle and return. (b) Toe raise. With the barbell in position as for squats, place the balls of the feet on a board about two inches high so that the heels are off the board. Rise up on the toes as far as possible, then lower the heels to the floor.

bouncing is counterproductive, and may lead to injury. Stretch slowly and methodically, taking plenty of time; repeat two or three times.

Leg stretches are useful for people who spend much of their time sitting, which results in a passive shortening of the muscles at the backs of the legs. Figure 5.6 illustrates two stretches that will lengthen lower leg muscles.

Rotating your arms at the shoulder joints is another good flexibility exercise. Ten to 15 arm circles each day can help you maintain full range of motion (Figure 5.7).

Increasing your aerobic endurance

Aerobic endurance: This term is synonymous with aerobic capacity, maximal aerobic power, or $\dot{V}_{O_2}$ max.

Although **aerobic endurance** or aerobic capacity is the last aspect of fitness we will discuss, it is extremely important. As we have mentioned several times previously, $\dot{V}_{O_2}$ max is an indicator of metabolic, respiratory, and circulatory capacity. Since $\dot{V}_{O_2}$ max depends on so many physiological functions, it is probably the best single indicator of physical fitness.

When you train to increase your aerobic capacity you improve both your respiratory and cardiovascular reserves. You also improve the metabolic capabilities of the muscles involved. Probably the most obvious change that you will notice is that you can perform longer and

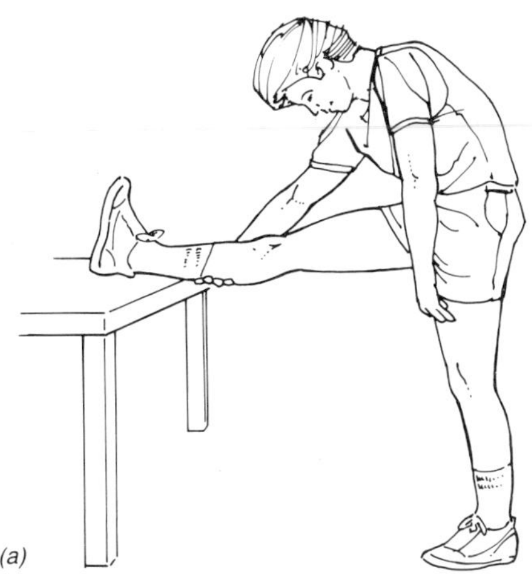
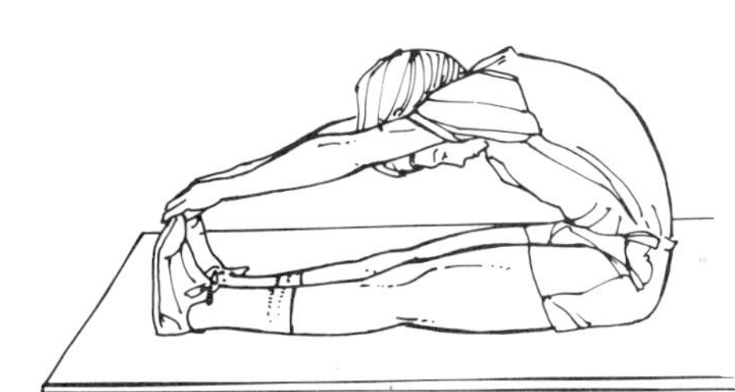

Figure 5.5 Flexibility exercises for the legs, hips, and back. Each of these exercises, done slowly two or three times daily, contributes to flexibility. (a) Hurdle stretch. Extend leg on support and attempt to touch forehead to knee; repeat with other leg. This stretches the hamstring muscles on the back of the thigh and the lower back muscles. (b) Toe touch. Sit with straight legs and attempt to touch toes with fingers. This stretches hamstring and lower back muscles.

with less apparent effort at endurance activities as your $\dot{V}_{O_2}$ max increases. You can climb an extra flight or two of stairs before you feel "winded," or you may feel as though you could keep running for another mile or two after you have covered your usual route.

Aerobic endurance activities   Programs to increase aerobic capacity should involve activities that: (1) use large muscle groups, (2) are done rhythmically, and (3) can be continued for at least 15 minutes at a time. There are many types of aerobic exercise that meet these qualifications: walking, jogging, running, swimming, bicycling, cross-country skiing, skating, rowing, rope skipping, and aerobic dancing are common examples.

Some activities include periods of aerobic effort, interspersed with anaerobic activity and/or rest; soccer, basketball, tennis, squash, racketball, hockey, and wrestling are examples. These activities can also have aerobic benefit, although it is more difficult to estimate how much improvement you will realize, since an unpredictable proportion of the activity is aerobic.

But whatever you choose as your conditioning activity, make sure it is fun enough for you to be faithful in doing it, and feasible for you to do often. It doesn't make sense to choose an activity for regular exercise that you cannot do in bad weather, or that requires you to go to a distant special facility, or that is too expensive for you to do regularly. Probably the very most important factor is that you should like what you choose to do; even if it is not ideal in terms of fitness

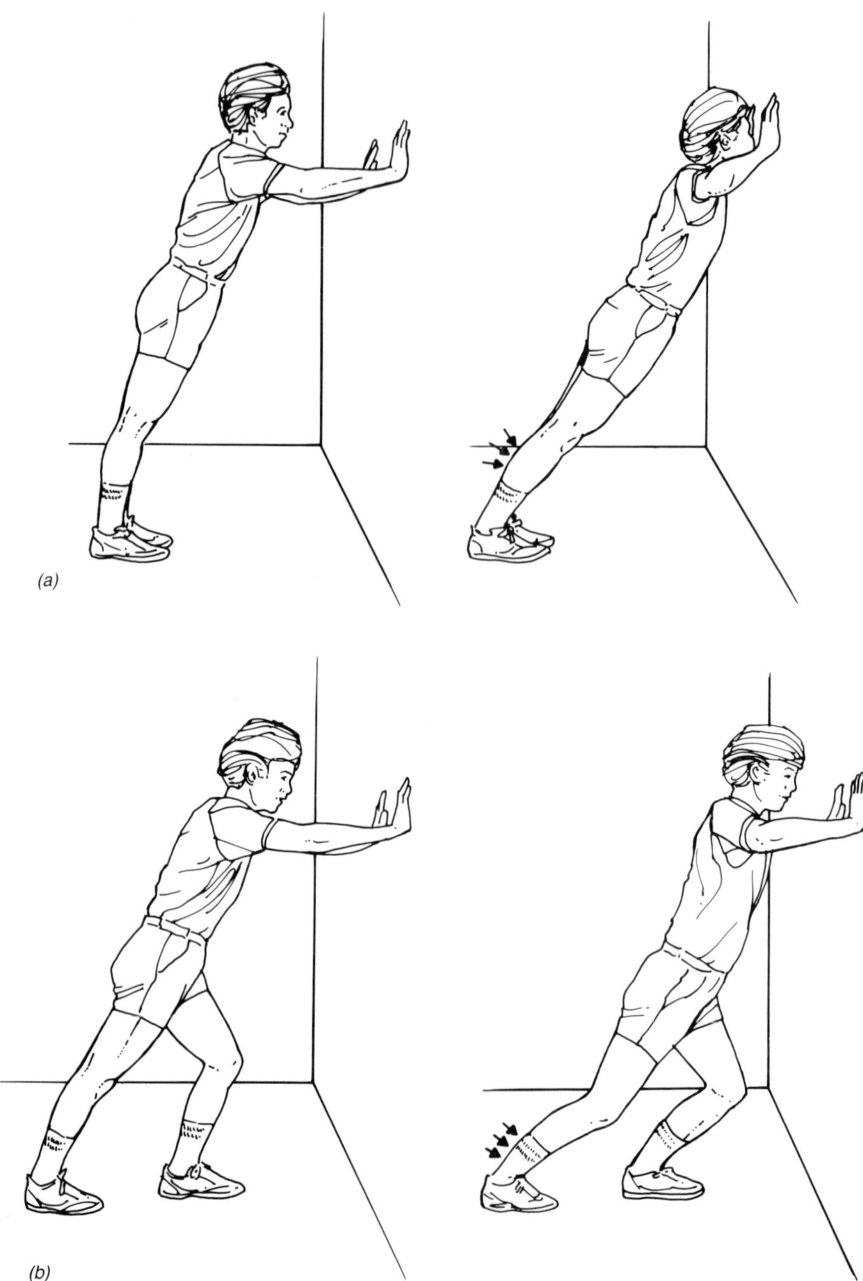

Figure 5.6 Stretching exercises for the muscles at the back of the lower leg. Use a wall for support to stretch the calf muscles. (a) While maintaining foot position and straight legs, flex arms and lean toward the wall. (b) Another version has you alternate one-leg stretches while flexing at knee and hip. Again, foot position is maintained.

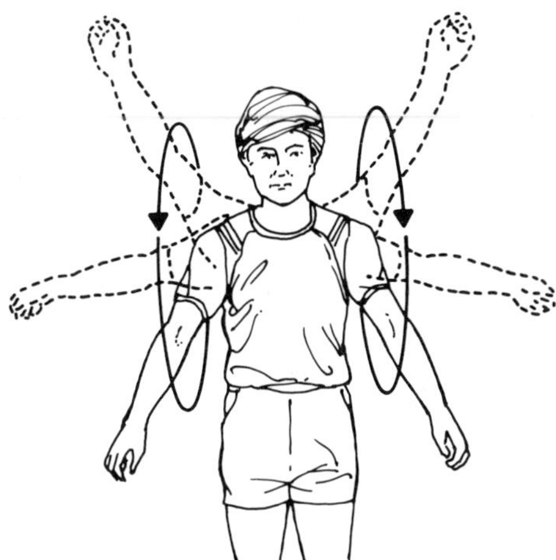

Figure 5.7 Flexibility exercises for the shoulders. Rotating your arms slowly in full circles, emphasizing extended range of motion, can help maintain full range of motion of the shoulder joints. Do 10 to 15 circles forward and then repeat backward.

benefits, doing it regularly will reap more benefits for you than an ideal program that you don't do very often.

Exercise time and frequency   The recommended duration and frequency of exercise for developing and maintaining fitness is 15 to 60 minutes of continuous aerobic activity three to five times per week. These are the recommendations of the American College of Sports Medicine (1978), the professional group concerned with exercise physiology, sports nutrition, and sports medicine.

You can decide how long to exercise within that broad recommended range by considering the intensity of the activity you have chosen: activities of lower intensity should be continued for a longer period of time. Generally speaking, it is better to exercise at a lower intensity for a longer period than to engage in very brief, extremely high intensity exercise; this is because there are more potential problems and a higher dropout rate associated with very high intensity programs.

In practical terms, many people find that it works well for them to exercise aerobically for a half hour every other day. This allows most people to fit the workouts into their schedules.

How hard should you push yourself?   We have already directed you toward the activities that can help you increase aerobic capacity. But since these activities can be done at different intensities, how can you tell when you're working hard enough to do yourself some good?

Measuring *heart rate* will give you the best guidance in this matter. You can easily feel your pulse in the arteries of the neck (the carotid arteries) that are on both sides of your trachea or windpipe; press the

Resting heart rate: Pulse count taken before exercise, standing quietly.

Maximal heart rate: Pulse taken when exercising intensely.

Training heart rate: Heart rate at which improvement in aerobic capacity is possible; the range of 60 to 90 percent of heart rate reserve added to resting heart rate.

tips of your fingers gently along either side of your windpipe under your jaw to find the pulsations (Figure 5.8). Count your pulse for 10 seconds; multiply by 6 to get your heart rate in beats/minute.

Determine your **resting heart rate** by taking your pulse when you are standing quietly before you exercise. You also need to know your **maximal heart rate**; you can determine it by taking your pulse after exercising as hard as possible for several minutes, or you can easily estimate it by subtracting your age from the number 220.

Next, substract your resting heart rate from your maximal heart rate; this difference is your heart rate reserve. Studies have shown that the minimal threshold for improving aerobic capacity is approximately 60 percent of the heart rate reserve above your resting heart rate. Therefore you should calculate what 60 percent of the heart rate reserve is, and add this figure to your resting heart rate; this gives you your (minimal) **training heart rate**, the lowest heart rate at which you are likely to improve aerobic capacity.

Exercise physiologists also suggest an upper limit that you should not exceed during aerobic activity; generally you should not exercise above 90 percent of your heart rate reserve (80 percent for a poorly conditioned person). The range between 60 and 90 percent represents the intensity at which you maintain and increase your aerobic capacity.

Self-check 5.1 will help you calculate your own training heart rate. Figure 5.9 is an example of how a young woman used the self-check to determine her training heart rate.

Certain environmental conditions can influence your heart rate. High heat and humidity put stress on the cardiovascular system to increase the blood supply to the skin surface for cooling. Therefore, while doing

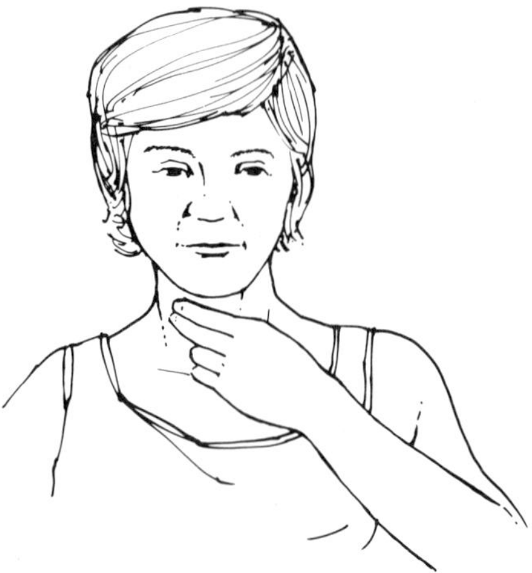

Figure 5.8   Finding your pulse. A convenient place to feel the pulsations of your heartbeat is in the carotid arteries next to your trachea (windpipe). Count the beats for 10 seconds and multiply by six to get your heart rate per minute.

Self-check 5.1   Determining your training heart rate range

1. Calculate your maximal heart rate (beats per minute) by subtracting your age from 220   1. _______ bpm
2. Take your resting heart rate   2. _______ bpm
3. Calculate your heart rate reserve by subtracting your resting heart rate (line 2) from your maximal heart rate (line 1)   3. _______ bpm
4. Calculate 60% of your heart rate reserve   4. _______ bpm
5. To determine your minimal training heart rate, add line 4 to your resting heart rate (line 2)   5. _______ bpm
6. Next calculate 90% of your heart rate reserve   6. _______ bpm
7. To determine your maximal training heart rate, add line 6 to your resting heart rate   7. _______ bpm
8. Record the range below, using the values from lines 5 and 7

Training heart rate range: from _______ bpm to _______ bpm.

Figure 5.9   A filled-in example of Self-check 5.1 for determining training heart rate range. This example is for Ellen, who is 21 years old and has a resting heart rate of 64 beats per minute (bpm).

1. Calculate your maximal heart rate (beats per minute) by subtracting your age from 220   1. _199_ bpm
2. Take your resting heart rate   2. _64_ bpm
3. Calculate your heart rate reserve by subtracting your resting heart rate (line 2) from your maximal heart rate (line 1)   3. _135_ bpm
4. Calculate 60% of your heart rate reserve   4. _81.0_ bpm
5. To determine your minimal training heart rate, add line 4 to your resting heart rate (line 2)   5. _145_ bpm
6. Next calculate 90% of your heart rate reserve   6. _121.5_ bpm
7. To determine your maximal training heart rate, add line 6 to your resting heart rate   7. _186_ bpm
8. Record the range below, using the values from lines 5 and 7

Training heart rate range: from _145_ bpm to _186_ bpm.

any given exercise in high heat and/or humidity, your heart rate will be higher; you need to lower the intensity of your exercise at those times to keep your heart rate within recommended training levels.

Designing an exercise program

To illustrate how to structure an exercise program, we will use the example of a walking and jogging program, since it is a form of exercise that can be done by almost everybody with a minimum of special equipment and in many different settings. We realize, though, that running is not for everyone; if it does not appeal to you, think of this description only as an example, and use it as a prototype for a program of aerobic activity of your choice.

The first five to seven minutes of every exercise session should be spent in **warm-up activity** that stretches your muscles (especially those you will be using in your chosen aerobic exercise) over their full range, and raises muscle temperature to the level that promotes optimal function.

Warm-up activity: Exercise that beneficially warms and stretches muscles in preparation for more intense activity.

For jogging (or any other exercise in which you support your weight with your legs) appropriate warm-up involves stretching the muscles of the calf (at the back of the leg between the knee and the ankle) and the hamstrings (at the back of the thigh). Refer back to Figure 5.5 and Figure 5.6 for these exercises. This warm-up is not only important for protecting you from injury during the subsequent aerobic exercise, but can also serve as some of the flexibility exercises recommended in any fitness program. In addition, include some arm circles (see Figure 5.7), which can help in loosening your arms and shoulders before you begin the aerobic part of your workout.

Once you have warmed up, you are ready for the aerobic exercise itself. Table 5.1 offers three programs for walking/jogging/running activities. Program Red is an appropriate beginning level for people who have been quite inactive; Program Blue is suitable for those accustomed to some activity but who are not well trained; and Program White is for those who have already been jogging regularly. Although those descriptions will help you decide which program to try first, check it for appropriateness by determining whether the activity brings you within your training heart rate range, and makes you feel slightly pushed but not overly stressed.

Each program has four to five phases; when one phase becomes too easy, move on to the next. You can evaluate this according to your heart rate: as you do your exercise program over days and weeks, your heart rate will gradually decline for any given pace, which is an effect of training. When your pulse falls below your training heart rate, you know it is time to advance to the next phase. After you have finished with the last phase of a given program, move to the first phase of the next-most-difficult program. The last phase of Program White can be used as an ongoing program for maintaining aerobic capacity.

Figure 5.10 shows how an individual's heart rate will change during an appropriate exercise session.

Cool-down period: Time after vigorous exercise in which warm-up activity is repeated.

Note that the last part of a workout should be a **cool-down period**. This routine is a repeat of the warm-up; it allows for a gradual, rather than abrupt, slowing down of your circulatory activity, and serves to relieve the tension which builds up in the lower back muscles, hamstrings, arms, and shoulders during jogging. In addition, flexibility ex-

Table 5.1   Three prescribed jogging programs

	Phase				
	I	II	III	IV	V
Program Red					
Stretch	5 min	5 min	5 min	5 min	5 min
Walk	4 min (120 steps/min)	3 min	2 min	1 min	—
Jog	1 min (5 mph)	2 min	3 min	4 min	36 min
	Repeat walk and jog 5×	Repeat walk and jog 5×	Repeat walk and jog 6×	Repeat walk and jog 6×	
Distance	1.4 miles	1.6 miles	2.1 miles	2.3 miles	2.3 miles
Cool-down	5 min	5 min	5 min	5 min	5 min
Total time	35 minutes	35 minutes	40 minutes	40 minutes	46 minutes
Program Blue					
Stretch	5 min	5 min	5 min	5 min	
Walk	2 min (134 steps/min)	1 min	½ min	—	
Jog	2 min (6 mph)	3 min	4 min	30 min	
	Repeat walk and jog 6×	Repeat walk and jog 7×	Repeat walk and jog 7×		
Distance	2 miles	2.6 miles	3.0 miles	3.0 miles	
Cool-down	5 min	5 min	5 min	5 min	
Total time	34 minutes	38 minutes	39 minutes	40 minutes	
Program White					
Stretch	5 min	5 min	5 min	5 min	
Pace	10 min/mile	9–9½ min/mile	8–8½ min/mile	7–7½ min/mile	
Distance	3 miles	3 miles	3 miles	3 miles	
Cool-down	5 min	5 min	5 min	5 min	
Total time	40 min	37–38½ min	34–35½ min	31–33½ min	

ercises may reduce residual muscle soreness. The cool-down period also offers an opportunity for additional flexibility exercises.

You can see from this walk/jog/run program that once you have found your beginning level, you should progress in small increments that keep your pulse within your recommended training range. You can structure a similar graduated program for any aerobic activity.

A key part of the whole experience is for exercise to be pleasant; don't make it another stressful event in your life. You will progress— relax and enjoy it!

According to opinion surveys, Americans seem to know that exercise is important to health. Yet, one-fourth to one-half of us do not do any deliberate exercise; and if you add those who exercise only occasionally,

Sticking With It

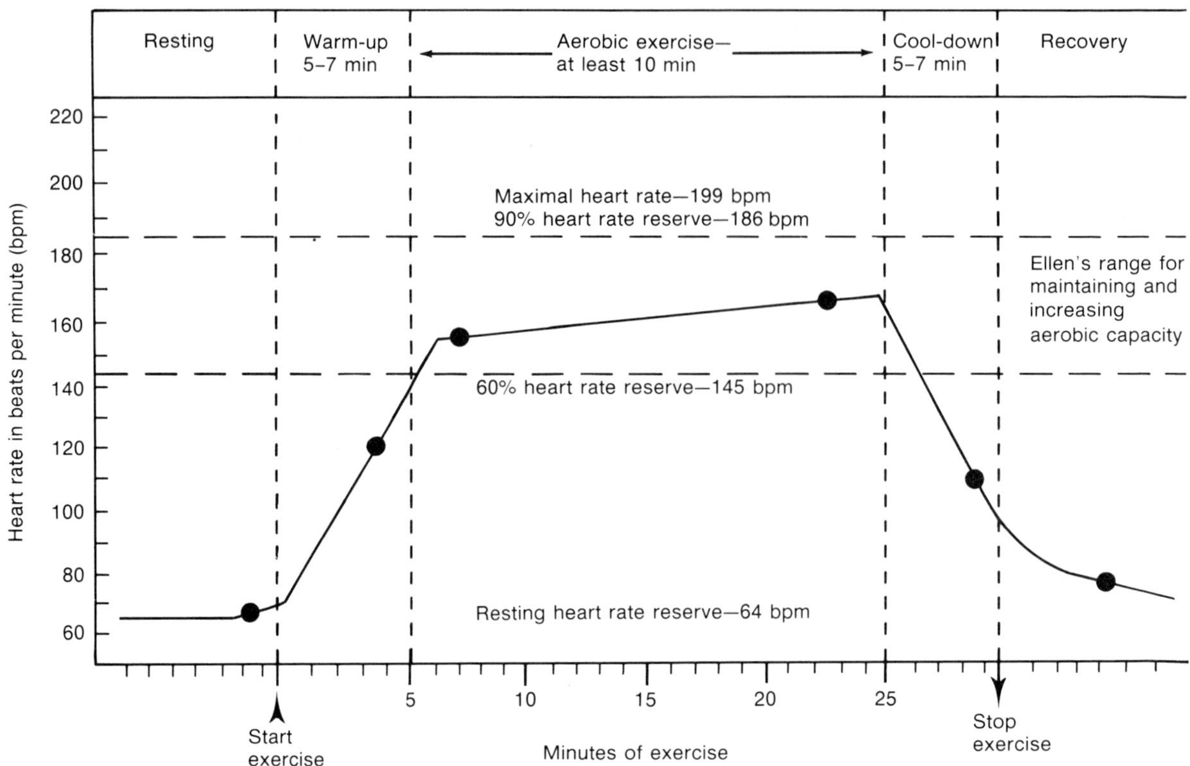

Figure 5.10 Changes in heart rate during an exercise session. This example uses the values determined for Ellen in Figure 5.9.

two-thirds of Americans do not exercise on a regular basis. Further, studies show that almost half the people who join an exercise program drop out in three to six months. Obviously, many people resist exercising regularly. Some behavioral psychologists have begun to study the factors that cause people to attend and adhere to exercise programs. The following suggestions are based on the work of these psychologists.

Motivating yourself

A behavioral tendency that seems to correlate with adherence is self-motivation: if you are a self-starter who does well at encouraging and praising yourself, you are more likely to stay with your program. In behavioral terms, you will probably succeed if you can give yourself energizing cues to exercise, and also have the ability to generate your own positive reinforcement, especially in the face of adversity.

On the other hand, if you know that you do not motivate yourself well, it may benefit you substantially to join a group program that is led by someone who can help motivate you. If you can talk to the leader of a program before you register for it, you may get a sense of whether the person could help you stay involved.

Gaining positive reinforcement

Most people find it helpful to get encouragement from others when they begin to exercise. Tell your roommate, family, and friends that you are starting a program. Especially tell those who are proponents of exercise, or who have a vested interest in the benefits you will get from the activity. If your roommate wishes you had the stamina to play an entire tennis match, he or she is likely to encourage you in your conditioning efforts. If your wife is worried about your high blood pressure, she is likely to be supportive of your exercise program.

Because positive reinforcement is so useful in helping people continue their exercise practices, you should learn to give yourself a generous amount of praise as well. Be lavish in your positive self-talk. Internalize the best of the praise you get from others; do it regularly for yourself, and you will become less dependent on others for their encouragement.

Exercising with a group

Another way to get positive reinforcement for your exercise efforts is to work out with a group. There is some evidence that people who exercise in a group have a higher adherence rate than people who exercise alone.

That is not to say that group exercise is the answer for everybody. Remember that positive reinforcers vary from person to person. Ask yourself whether social encouragement and praise are important for you. If so, a group program is more likely to keep you exercising.

Not only do the participants encourage each other, but the leader can also be very influential, especially when he or she gives individual encouragement and praise about the participants' progress. A leader might jog next to you and comment on how you have picked up your pace since you started the program two weeks ago, or ask you how much easier it seems now than when you began. This is much more likely to keep people involved than when a leader gives feedback to the group as a whole; a general announcement of, "You're really doing great, everybody," does not have the same value.

However, if you're a person who does not benefit much from the praise of others, a group program will not particularly help keep you exercising.

Using response cost

Especially at the beginning of a group or individual program, it might be helpful to employ the principle of response cost. That is, put something you value at stake; if you fail to adhere to your program, you lose the item.

In some group programs, each participant puts up a certain amount of money; at the end of the program, the money is shared among those who have attended the required number of sessions. If you are exercising alone, deposit a significant amount of money with a friend. If you reach your exercise goals you get the money back; if not, the money is given, as previously decided, to a favorite charity. This technique can be helpful for getting a person "over the hump" at the beginning of a program.

Structuring your own program

Many of the factors found to be related to exercise adherence involve the planning and implementation steps of the behavior modification process. For example, it is important for people to design the steps of their own program; this enhances continuation. In other words, even after you have determined what form of exercise you want to do to improve your fitness, you should be the one who decides when you will increase the intensity of the activity, how long each session will be, and how many times each week you will do it. Of course, you should bear in mind the minimum amount of exercise required for achieving and maintaining fitness.

You need to be responsive to your own ability level and rate of progress. Applying a program to yourself that has been perfect for somebody else may be a disaster; if it's too slow for you, you may become bored with it; or if it's too fast, you may become frustrated that you cannot keep up.

This need for individual pacing holds true even if you are part of a group program. Avoid programs in which all members exercise in lockstep with each other. Look for those that permit flexibility and individualization.

Thinking about the right things

You may be able to improve your chances of sticking with your conditioning program by having your mind on the right kinds of things while you are exercising.

There are two general kinds of thought pattern—association and dissociation. **Association** means that you concentrate on your activity and your body's responses to it; **dissociation** means that you think about things other than what you are doing and how your body feels. There is evidence that for the beginning exerciser, it is helpful to use dissociation strategies; that is, distract yourself from how you feel by thinking about almost anything else.

Especially for somebody who has been habitually inactive, starting an exercise program involves certain discomforts; but if a person uses such ploys as recalling a favorite movie, enjoying the scenery, or chatting with a friend, he or she can often get beyond the minor physical complaints to the point where positive reinforcers, such as feeling healthier and looking better, begin to maintain and increase exercise.

However, you must be cautious about using dissociation. First of all, pain is the body's signal that it is being stressed more than normally.

Association: Thinking about what you are doing and how your body is responding to it.

Dissociation: Thinking about something other than what you are doing physically and how your body is responding to it.

Certainly, severe pain is a message that you should stop or ease up on what you are doing. But a small amount of extra stress is needed to bring about improvement in fitness, and it will probably be accompanied by minor pain. How can you discriminate between this "harmless" pain and "danger-signal" pain?

If a minor pain persists or gets worse, you should respond to the message by discontinuing the stress on that part of your body. Either cut back your exercise intensity to a level that is not painful, or quit for the day. After you have exercised for a few sessions, you will begin to recognize the difference between the indicators that you are exercising at an appropriate level for improving your fitness and those that say you're at risk of injuring yourself.

Of course, if you have a chronic disease or disability, listening to your body messages and responding appropriately is a very important way of heading off trouble. You should not use dissociation; only healthy people should employ it.

Another note about dissociation: experienced athletes do not use it. From long experience, they know that it is to their advantage to "read" their bodies and modify their activities in order to give the best performance they can at any given moment. Using *association* is smart for people at such high levels of performance, whereas using *dissociation* has utility for the beginner.

Practicing relapse prevention

Relapse prevention is another useful adjunct to a program: it emphasizes that the issue is not *whether* a person will periodically miss a few sessions, but *how* he or she will deal with this situation *when* it happens. Relapse prevention requires you to think ahead to situations in which you might fail to exercise for a time—such as when you get sick, are out of town, or have to study for exams—and then to envision how to begin your program again. The idea is to prevent *missing* from becoming *quitting*.

Relapse prevention: Planning ways to restart your exercise program after missing a few sessions.

Some methods to try are the following:

1. You might think about calling somebody with whom you have exercised, and making arrangements to go with that person the next day.
2. You could imagine talking with your friends about your intentions to get back to your program.
3. You could plan to resume your exercise at a level that was slightly less challenging than the level at which you stopped; this would accommodate to some lost capacity.
4. You could encourage yourself with the reminder that you can regain whatever you lost.

Mentally preparing in such ways for some inevitable lapses helps keep a person from catastrophizing, such as thinking, "Now that I've missed two weeks, I've blown it. I'll never be able to get back to it again.''

In this chapter we have described how to set up your own individualized exercise program, and have given you some tips on how to keep yourself at it. This may be all that you need. However, for many activities you may need special equipment and you may also have to consider your environment.

These topics will be discussed in the next chapter, Chapter 6.

Exercise Environment and Equipment 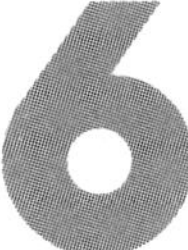

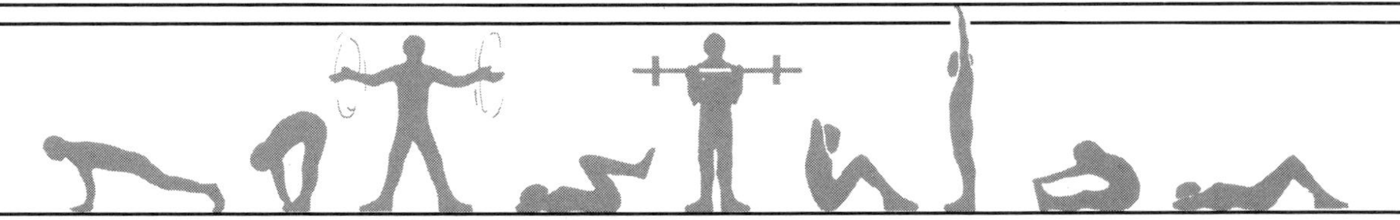

Outline

In the two preceding chapters we have dealt mainly with *the body* and exercise. Now it's time to focus on some *external factors*—the environment and various types of equipment.

If you exercise outdoors, you know what a difference the weather can make in your enjoyment of an activity. A soccer game played on a dry day when the temperature is 55°F, feels quite different from one played when it is humid and 80°F. A tennis match attempted in a 25 mph wind on a 45°F day is likely to be far less pleasant than one played when the air is still and the temperature is 60°F.

   But even more critical than their effects on enjoyment, these factors of environmental temperature, humidity, and wind can have a major

Allow for the Weather

impact on your physical well-being during exercise. They can affect your whole body and its ability to function.

One way that is sometimes used to avoid the vagaries of the weather is to move activities into climate-controlled facilities. However, that approach is not practical for all sports, and is usually very expensive; furthermore, it takes away the considerable pleasure that being outdoors sometimes offers. Therefore, it is important to learn how to adapt to weather conditions so that you can safely exercise outside.

The major physiological concerns are the maintenance of normal internal temperature and **hydration** (body-water status). If either factor is substantially raised or lowered, problems may arise. Your metabolism will become less efficient, performance will progressively deteriorate, structural damage may result, and if the situation continues to worsen, ultimately death will occur.

Normal **core** (internal) temperature is 98.6°F, give or take a degree either way, for individual variation. A person is at risk of death when his or her internal temperature drops to approximately 80°F (although a few have survived lower temperatures), or if it rises above approximately 108°F. Low body temperature is called **hypothermia**; excessively high temperature is called **hyperthermia**.

As far as hydration is concerned, the body of a normal-weight adult is approximately 60 percent water by weight (although we often get fatter and consequently relatively drier as we age). Deterioration of physical performance occurs when as little as 3 percent of body weight is lost as water, and death occurs at about a 12 percent water loss. There is little risk from overconsumption of fluids; you would have to consume gallons more fluid than you actually need in a day to cause death.

Fortunately, the body has mechanisms that help maintain internal temperature and hydration at normal levels. Before we discuss how environmental factors can influence body temperature and water content, we will provide some background regarding these regulatory mechanisms. Since there is considerable interaction between internal and environmental factors, this distinction is somewhat artificial.

Physiological factors control temperature and hydration

The body has various ways of producing, conserving, and dissipating heat and water in order to maintain normal temperature.

Most body heat is produced by the processes that keep you alive (such as heartbeat, breathing, etc.), which collectively are called your **resting or basal metabolism**. Your resting metabolism produces sufficient heat to keep your body temperature around 98.6°F. A small amount of additional heat is produced when your body digests, absorbs, and metabolizes food; this is called the **specific dynamic effect**.

Physical activity is the third source of heat produced by the body; it causes body temperature to rise above its normal rest level. After just a few minutes of exercise, your body reaches a new temperature

---

Hydration: The level of water present in the body.

Core: The interior of the body.

Hypothermia: Abnormally low body temperature.

Hyperthermia: Abnormally high body temperature.

Resting or basal metabolism: The energy expended (or oxygen consumed) during a period of physical, emotional, and digestive rest.

Specific dynamic effect: The energy used for digesting, absorbing and metabolizing food that has been consumed.

which it maintains as long as you continue exercising at that intensity. Figure 6.1 shows how body temperature increases proportionately with oxygen uptake or exercise intensity.

As internal temperature begins to rise, body mechanisms for dissipating surplus heat start functioning. Blood vessels near the skin surface dilate so that blood flow to the skin is increased, and heat is lost from the skin surface. You see evidence of this increased blood supply when you are "flushed." If this blood flow to the skin gets very high, you probably will not be able to perform at your best, because your muscles receive less blood—and therefore less oxygen and nutrients that they need to produce energy. On the other hand, if your internal temperature decreases from a normal rest level, the blood vessels near the skin constrict, and the blood supply is concentrated in the body's core. There, the blood does not lose heat as rapidly because of the insulation the body tissues provide.

In addition, when body temperature rises, sweating occurs, and the **evaporation** of sweat from the skin reduces body temperature. Your body can secrete as much as three liters of sweat in an hour or two of strenuous exercise; the evaporation of each liter from the skin removes almost 600 kcalories of heat from the body, leaving the skin cooler. This allows for a shift of more heat from the interior to the skin.

Note that it is the *evaporation process, not the perspiration itself*, that helps cool you. Sweat which drips off your body or is trapped in clothing is not evaporated and therefore does not result in body-heat

Evaporation: The transfer of heat by the vaporization of water (sweat).

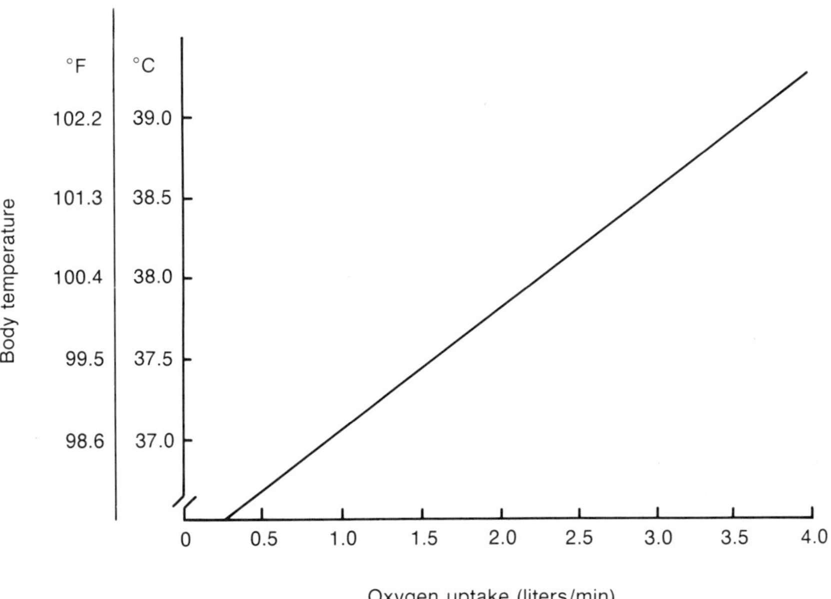

Figure 6.1   The harder you exercise, the warmer you get. This illustration shows that body temperature is directly related to oxygen uptake and therefore to exercise intensity.

loss. This explains the oppressive feeling you may notice on humid or "muggy" days; if the air around you already contains a lot of moisture, less evaporation occurs, and you retain more body heat. It also explains why clothing which interferes with evaporation, such as rubber suits or clothes of tightly constructed synthetic materials, make you hot. Expecially if such garments fit close to the body, they confine the heat and sweat around you, reduce evaporation, and may cause body temperature to rise to a dangerously high level. We will discuss appropriate clothing later in this chapter.

When you perspire heavily, your body conserves some water by producing less urine. This occurs because a large portion of your blood supply is directed to muscle and skin, and less is channeled through the kidneys. However, reduced urine production during heavy sweating can only partly compensate for the large volume of fluid lost as sweat.

Weather conditions influence body temperature and hydration

Environmental factors can add or remove heat from the body, as well as influence hydration status.

Conduction: The transfer of heat by direct contact with another substance.

Air temperature   **Conduction** of heat between the air and the body can lead to losses or gains in body heat. However, since air is a poor conductor of heat, it is not an important medium for dissipating surplus body heat unless the air is considerably cooler than you are.

Humidity   As explained earlier, high humidity interferes with the evaporation of perspiration. If you become overheated and begin to perspire on a humid day, your sweat will not evaporate and cool you. Consequently you will continue to sweat without obtaining relief. Very low humidity increases evaporation, even if you are not obviously sweating. Therefore both extremes of humidity can have a dehydrating effect.

Radiation: The transfer of heat by way of electro-magnetic waves.

Sun   **Radiation** from the sun is another factor that can increase body temperature. It can substantially add to the heat load imposed on a person who is exercising on a hot day. Clothing or shade of any origin can effectively shield you. Light-colored clothing reflects the sun's rays and reduces body heat gain.

Relative wind velocity   Relative wind velocity measures the movement of air over the body surface. If you are not moving or are moving slowly, the relative wind velocity is close to the reported wind velocity. If the air is calm and you are running at 8 mph, the relative wind velocity is 8 mph.

If the air is hotter than your body surface, movement of air across the body will tend to raise your temperature; but if the air temperature is lower than body temperature, movement promotes body heat loss.

This is the basis for the wind-chill factor given in weather reports. It also explains why, on a calm day, a person loses heat faster while riding a bicycle than walking, even though the intensity of the two activities may not be much different.

Moving air can also influence your hydration status by affecting the rate of evaporation of moisture from your skin surface. On a windy day—especially a dry one—your body loses considerable fluid. If it is also hot and you are exercising, fluid losses can be so large as to be dangerous.

Preventing hyperthermia and dehydration

There are several measures you can take to help reduce your risk of hyperthermia and dehydration.

Be cautious of high temperature and humidity   Figure 6.2 will help you judge when heat and humidity are so high that exercise may be dangerous. When conditions fall in the *danger zone*, shorten your exercise period. When temperature and humidity are in the *cancel zone*, it is wise to postpone exercise until conditions are not as severe; for example, temperatures may be lower in the evening or early morning.

Drink enough water   At any temperature, it is important to drink water before, during, and after you exercise. Your sense of thirst may not prompt you to drink enough to maintain normal hydration, so drink more than you are thirsty for (see Table 6.1). This becomes increasingly critical as the air temperature rises, and the longer you exercise.

Some people suggest adding salt and/or sugar to the water, but neither has been shown to be superior to plain water. In fact, adding such substances may delay absorption of the water, and usually neither

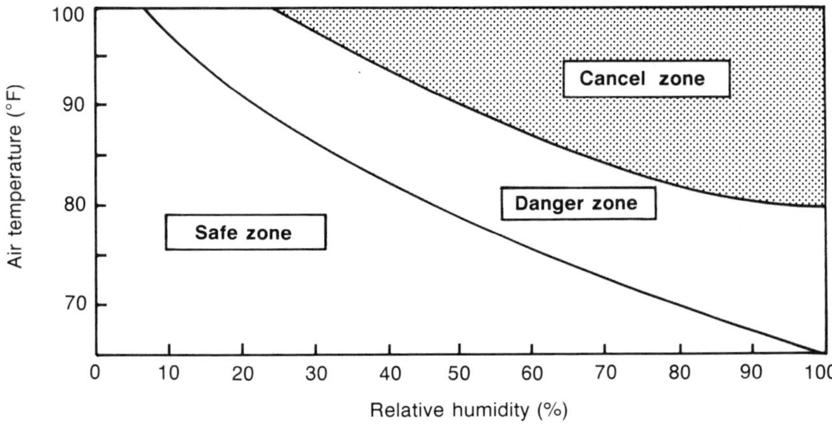

Figure 6.2   The effect of temperature and humidity on exercise safety. Certain temperature and humidity combinations are hazardous to your health; make sure it's safe to exercise.

Table 6.1   Guidelines for adequate water consumption

When to drink water	Amount
Before activity	
2 hours before	2 to 3 cups
10–15 minutes before	2 cups
During activity	
Every 10–15 minutes	1/2 to 1 cup
After activity	
Every 15–30 minutes, until pre-exercise weight is regained (2 cups/lb lost)	1 cup each time

salt nor sugar is needed during recreational exercise. Requirements for salt and sugar during endurance activities will be discussed later in the chapters on nutrition.

There is some debate about whether the water consumed during exercise should be cold or at room temperature. Cold water can lower the internal temperature slightly when it comes in contact with body fluids and tissues; this is a benefit. Also, there is evidence that cold water is absorbed more rapidly. On the other hand, cold water taken *after* strenuous exercise in the heat may cause stomach cramps. Even though there is no clear-cut answer as to what temperature of water is best, all experts agree that you need to drink water, and plenty of it.

Wear suitable clothing   The clothing you wear can also help you avoid hyperthermia. The guidelines are simple:

- . Wear as little clothing as is socially acceptable unless exercising in the sun, when you should wear light colors to reflect the heat.
- Choose lightweight and loosely woven garments to enhance evaporation.

Acclimatize yourself   If you exercise in high heat and humidity for an hour or two each day, after approximately one week your body will have made some limited adaptations to those conditions. It may initially be necessary to exercise at a lower intensity, however. Such **acclimatization** occurs spontaneously in people who regularly exercise outdoors as seasonal temperatures rise. This principle can also be deliberately applied when a person prepares for competition in a warmer climate.

Compared to an unacclimatized person, an acclimatized person will not get as hot at the same exercise intensity; will have an increased ability to sweat; and will have sweat that is not as salty. A fitter individual will acclimatize more rapidly and maintain a lower body temperature for the same exercise intensity than a less fit person.

Acclimatization: Adaptation to a change in the environment, such as heat or altitude.

In addition, during the acclimatization period all safeguards, such as consuming adequate water, must also be practiced.

Treating emergencies   Although prevention is the best method, emergency situations may arise nonetheless. *Heat cramps, heat exhaustion,* and *heat stroke* are increasingly serious forms of hyperthermia, all of which require intervention. The worst of them, heat stroke, may result in death if not promptly treated.

Table 6.2 describes these conditions and their symptoms, and indicates appropriate treatment for each one. You should become familiar with these symptoms so that if you experience them you will realize that you need to drink water and cool off. People who are responsible for the welfare of others—such as teachers, coaches, and race organizers—should not only know the symptoms but should also be prepared to administer first aid and obtain emergency medical services as needed.

Table 6.2   Indications of and treatment for hyperthermia

	Symptoms	Weight loss	Treatment
Heat cramps	• Thirst • Chills • Clammy skin • Throbbing heartbeat • Nausea	Up to 5% of body weight as sweat • Up to 5 pounds for 100-pound athlete • Up to 7½ pounds for 150-pound athlete • Up to 10 pounds for 200-pound athlete	Athlete should: • Drink ½ cup of water every 10–15 minutes • During breaks—move to shade and remove as much clothing as possible
Heat exhaustion	• Reduced sweating • Dizziness • Headache • Shortness of breath • Weak, rapid pulse • Lack of saliva • Extreme fatigue	5–10% of body weight as sweat • 5–10 pounds for 100-pound athlete • 7½–15 pounds for 150-pound athlete • 10–20 pounds for 200-pound athlete	Athlete should: • Stop exercise and move to a cool environment • Drink 2 cups of water for every pound lost • Take off wet clothing and sit on a chair in a cold shower • Place an ice bag on his or her head
Heat stroke	• Lack of sweat • Dry, hot skin • Lack of urine • Hallucinations • Swollen tongue • Deafness • Visual disturbances • Aggression • Unsteady walking • Excessively high body temperature	Over 10 percent of body weight as sweat • Over 10 pounds for 100-pound athlete • Over 15 pounds for 150-pound athlete • Over 20 pounds for 200-pound athlete	You should: • Call for emergency medical treatment • Until help arrives, place ice bags on back and front of athlete's head • Remove clothing and rub alcohol over most of the athlete's body • Seat athlete on chair in cold shower

Despite the availability of such information, every year there are deaths caused by exercising in hot and humid conditions, especially during football practice. Such deaths are particularly sad because they are often easily preventable. By exercising at the prescribed training heart rate you reduce the chance of a heat-related injury. As heat and humidity levels increase, your exercise intensity must be decreased to remain at the training heart rate.

Environment influences body cooling and hydration

Generally, exercising in the cold presents fewer serious health problems than exercising in the heat. This is partly because activity generates considerable heat which counteracts the cold. However, under certain conditions hypothermia of the whole body or of some body parts may occur.

Air temperature   Hypothermia of the body core is usually preceded by shivering, numbness, and/or clumsiness. If you feel these symptoms, you will probably instinctively look for warm shelter to regain normal body temperature; for this reason low core temperature is not a common problem.

However, if a person is in an undeveloped or isolated area, core hypothermia is a greater risk. For example, if you are hiking alone in the mountains in winter, cross-country skiing alone in a remote area, or snowmobiling by yourself in an isolated place, you are inviting trouble. Although hiking and skiing usually produce sufficient heat to maintain normal body temperature, if you get lost, have an equipment problem, are injured, or become so fatigued that you can no longer keep moving, hypothermia may occur. Proper clothing and a friend might help you, but being sure that you are near warm shelter at all times is even more important.

The most common problem encountered during winter exercise is *frostbite*. The extremities of the body (arms and legs) can withstand a much wider range of temperatures than the body core. Although a very small drop in core temperature will produce shivering and severe discomfort that make you seek shelter, a decrease in the temperature of ears, hands, or toes does not send such strong messages. Rather, the body's response is to greatly reduce blood flow to these areas, which conserves heat in the body core but renders the extremities susceptible to frostbite. This can occur in a relatively short time—sometimes just minutes—depending on the air temperature and wind. The following are points to remember for the treatment of frostbite:

1. Obtain medical help if possible.
2. Thaw tissue but only when in a *sheltered* area so there is no danger of refreezing.
3. Immerse frozen area in water at 100 to 110°F, but no hotter.

4. Do not rub area, especially not with snow.
5. Avoid putting weight on frostbitten feet.
6. Don't put frostbitten part very close to a heat source.
7. Don't break or bandage blisters.

It is a common misconception that breathing cold winter air will harm the lungs or air passages. This concern is unfounded. For example, for a person resting at temperatures as low as $-25°F$, the inspired air will be warmed to more than $80°F$ by the time it reaches the trachea. There is no evidence that lung tissues are damaged even after a full day of exercise at subzero temperatures.

Humidity   As it does in the case of heat stress, humidity plays a large role in the body's response to cold. When the humidity is high, people feel colder than they do when the humidity is low. Another important factor to consider is that cold air contains less moisture than warm air; dehydration in cold weather may be a problem because the rate of evaporation increases in such dry air.

Relative wind velocity   Of greater significance in the cold than humidity, however, is the relative wind velocity. On a completely calm winter day, if you are on an iceboat moving at 50 miles per hour, the relative wind speed on your body is 50 mph even though there is no wind. This can chill you considerably beyond the effect of the air temperature.

Preventing hypothermia and dehydration
Just as there are guidelines for exercising in a hot environment, there are ways to play it smart and safe in the cold.

Respect the wind-chill factor   Table 6.3 shows what the equivalent temperatures are for various actual thermometer readings and estimated wind speeds. It shows which wind-chill levels indicate that there is little danger, increasing danger, or great danger. Respecting such indices can save you from hypothermia and even death.

Drink enough water   Drink ample fluids to avoid dehydration. Because you are not likely to get as thirsty when exercising in the cold as you do in the heat, you may forget to drink enough. Drink fluids even though you aren't thirsty.

Wear suitable clothing   Dressing properly is also very important in preventing hypothermia. Wearing several layers of clothing is usually more effective for maintaining body temperature than wearing heavy, bulky clothes. If you overheat during exercise and you are wearing layers, you can just remove one layer. If you are wearing bulky clothes,

Table 6.3 Wind-chill factor chart

Estimated wind speed (MPH)	Actual thermometer reading (°F)											
	50	40	30	20	10	0	−10	−20	−30	−40	−50	−60
	Wind-chill temperature (°F)											
Calm	50	40	30	20	10	0	−10	−20	−30	−40	−50	−60
5	48	37	27	16	6	−5	−15	−26	−36	−47	−57	−68
10	40	28	16	4	−9	−24	−33	−46	−58	−70	−83	−95
15	36	22	9	−5	−18	−32	−45	−58	−72	−85	−99	−112
20	32	18	4	−10	−25	−39	−53	−67	−82	−96	−110	−124
25	30	16	0	−15	−29	−44	−59	−74	−88	−104	−118	−133
30	28	13	−2	−18	−33	−48	−63	−79	−94	−109	−125	−140
35	27	11	−4	−20	−35	−51	−67	−82	−98	−113	−129	−145
40[a]	26	10	−6	−21	−37	−53	−69	−85	−100	−116	−132	−148

LITTLE DANGER (for properly clothed person).	INCREASING DANGER from freezing of exposed flesh	GREAT DANGER

[a]Wind speeds greater than 40 MPH have little additional effect.

you may not have that option; furthermore, such clothes may hinder your activity.

If you are overdressed, your body temperature will rise, you will perspire heavily, and the evaporation of sweat might result in chilling, particularly during periods when you decrease exercise intensity.

Proper clothing can facilitate sweat evaporation at high exercise intensities, and also can provide protection from the cold at low intensities. Clothing made of wool qualifies in both regards. Drops of perspiration that form on the skin are absorbed by wool fibers and are retained for some time so that they evaporate slowly, thus preventing rapid heat loss. Also, air is trapped among wool fibers, making wool a good insulator.

Clothing made of nylon and Gore-Tex provide protection against the wind. Gore-Tex offers the added benefit of allowing perspiration to pass through and evaporate while preventing rain from penetrating through it.

Many runners and skiers wear a layer of light cotton clothing next to the body for comfort, followed by a wool garment or sweatshirt, and finally a light-weight wind breaker of nylon or Gore-Tex. These layers are particularly useful for the upper body, since in running and skiing the chest bears the brunt of the wind, and thus is especially vulnerable to the cold.

Since the extremities are likely to become frostbitten, protect your hands with mittens, which are generally warmer than gloves. Two pairs of socks provide extra insulation for the feet. A hat will prevent excessive loss of heat from the head; ear muffs and ski goggles are also useful. In severe cold it may be necessary to cover the lower part of your face with a mask or a "sheik" veil. The latter does not inhibit breathing as much as a face mask does, yet provides some warmth and protection from wind.

Play It Smart in High Places

At high elevations, the air is usually quite dry. This in itself promotes faster evaporation of water from the body. In addition, more rapid breathing results in greater moisture loss from the lungs. Because of the additional increase in respiration rate while exercising, an individual can quickly become dehydrated. Therefore skiers, hikers, and others who are active at high altitudes need to drink extra fluids. People are often surprised to learn this, because they do not expect to need extra water in a cool environment.

Indoors at high altitudes the situation may be even more exaggerated. When cold, dry air is brought inside and heated, its relative humidity becomes even lower. Even when humidifiers are used, inside air may be so dry as to lead to skin cracking and nosebleeds.

Exposure to the sun may present another problem at high altitudes, especially for those who have not had much recent exposure. Especially in the spring, when the sun's rays are more direct than in winter and are intensified by reflection off the snow, due to the abundance of ultraviolet light skiers may receive serious burns and/or cold sores. Fortunately, good sun screens are now available which can alleviate these problems. The higher the number on the sun screen, the greater the effectiveness.

Another effect you are likely to notice when you are at a higher elevation than normal is that your ability to perform aerobic activities is lower than usual. This is due to the fact that at the lower atmospheric pressure characteristic of higher altitudes, less oxygen gets into your blood stream, and $\dot{V}_{O_2}$ max is lower. At elevations above 5,000 feet, a person's $\dot{V}_{O_2}$ max decreases by 3 percent for every additional 1,000 feet of altitude, with predictable negative effects on performance. Figure 6.3 shows this direct relationship between altitude and $\dot{V}_{O_2}$ max.

This is particularly significant for athletes; the issue received considerable attention in 1968 when the Olympic Games were held in Mexico City, which is at an elevation of approximately 7,500 feet. Athletes competing in *anaerobic* events did not need to take the altitude into account, but those involved in *aerobic* activities had to consider ways to minimize the inevitable deterioration in performance that occurs at such elevations.

Basically, they had two choices, neither of which would prove to be entirely satisfactory: to train at that altitude for approximately three weeks prior to the games to permit some acclimatization to occur, or to fly in on the day of competition. Anything in between carried a more severe penalty. The reasons are not totally clear, but for several

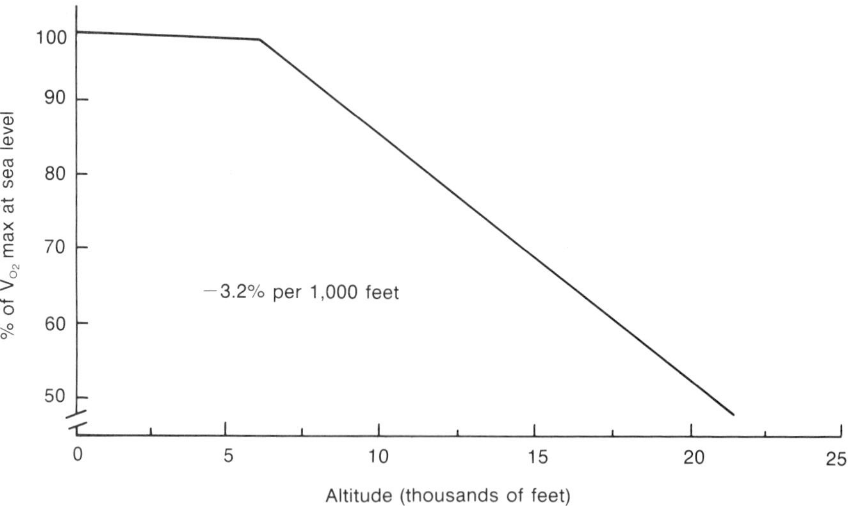

Figure 6.3 Decrease in $\dot{V}_{O_2}$ max at increasing altitudes. Note that oxygen uptake capacity remains at 100% at altitudes below 5,000 feet.

days after arrival at high altitude, performance progressively deteriorates before it slowly begins to improve. Of course, people who live for long periods at high altitudes eventually become totally adapted to their elevations.

Mountain sickness: Constellation of symptoms (headache, thirst, drowsiness, sleeplessness, nausea, loss of appetite) occurring in some people within one day of arrival at over 10,000 feet.

Some people are affected by **mountain sickness** when they ascend to altitudes above 10,000 feet. Anywhere from 2 to 14 hours after arrival they experience headache, thirst, drowsiness but inability to sleep, nausea, and loss of appetite. Generally these symptoms subside; if not, the best treatment is to return to lower altitude.

Pulmonary edema: Fluid accumulation in the lungs that can occur in some people within a few days of arrival at over 11,000 feet; requires emergency treatment.

A much more serious problem some people experience at elevations over 11,000 feet is **pulmonary edema** (fluid accumulation in the lungs) which is one form of mountain sickness and occurs 24 to 72 hours after arrival. This can be caused by pulmonary hypertension which forces fluid out of the blood into the space between the capillaries and the alveoli. Typical symptoms are severe dyspnea (shortness of breath) and coughing. The condition can be life-threatening. Emergency treatment includes administration of oxygen, and removal to a lower altitude as soon as possible.

Exercising in Neptune's World

Water is another popular environment for sports that has its own unique pleasures and risks. Water can conduct heat 20 times better than air; therefore, water that is cooler than body temperature readily removes body heat. This is why you feel very comfortable when exercising vigorously in water at 80°F, but you might feel unbearably hot doing the same intensity of exercise in 80°F air.

This attribute of water also has its dark side: cold water presents great risk. Every year there are many deaths from hypothermia resulting from submersion in cold water. In the case of prolonged exposure to cold water, being a good swimmer does not help.

Figure 6.4 gives estimated survival times in cold water. However, there are ways to safeguard against this risk when you use a boat in cold water.

Cold-water boating

You need to recognize the hazards and be cautious when boating on cold water. Rowing, kayaking, and canoeing are excellent forms of exercise, but are risky in cold water because these boats can easily tip over. Wearing a life vest (a personal flotation device, or PFD) at all times in such craft is absolutely imperative on cold water.

Boating is safer in narrow rivers than in lakes because of the proximity of the shore. However, if you fall overboard at a considerable distance from land, you can conserve body heat and energy if you remain with your boat, raise as much of your body out of the water as you can, and rest as much as possible.

Swimming

Swimming (in water of moderate temperature) is excellent exercise. Because of the buoyancy of the water, swimmers do not experience the forceful impact on the joints of the lower extremities that is pro-

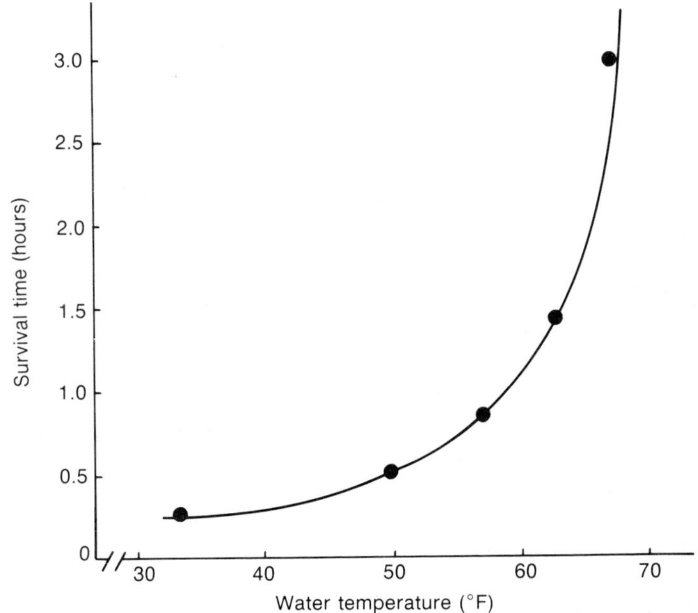

Figure 6.4   Estimated survival time in cold water.

duced by jogging and other weight-bearing forms of exercise. In this regard, swimming is a safer sport.

However, when the body is immersed in water, there is always risk of drowning. People should swim only either with a companion or when and where a qualified lifeguard is on duty, and observe any posted precautions for the area.

For people who swim underwater a lot, there are additional concerns. Swimming underwater results in greater-than-normal pressure on the body. Normal atmospheric pressure is about 14.7 pounds per square inch (psi); for each foot you dive below the surface, the weight of the water adds almost 0.5 psi. The increased pressure itself does not cause problems: your body can withstand enormous pressure if it is equalized inside and outside the body. It is the pressure *differential* between the inside and outside of the body which can be the source of problems.

For example, if you hold your breath as you dive to greater depth, a partial vacuum develops in the lungs, and blood or other fluid may leak in. Similarly, if the air pressure in the middle ear is lower than surrounding pressure, blood may be drawn into the middle ear, or the eardrum might rupture. Ear plugs are not recommended because the external pressure may force them deep into the ear canal.

As you descend, if you are wearing goggles, they may be sucked tighter on your face because of the increasing water pressure. Since air cannot be introduced into the space behind the goggles to lessen this pressure differential, bleeding from the vessels in the eyes or skin can occur. A face mask which goes over the nose also is preferable to goggles, because breathing into the mask can equalize the pressure.

The reverse problem occurs if you hold your breath while ascending from deep water. After you have swum for a while in deep water, the air in all cavities of your body—such as your lungs, sinuses, middle ear, intestines—becomes somewhat compressed from the water pressure. If you ascend rapidly, the water pressure on the outside of your body decreases rapidly, and your internal pressure is greater. As you rise toward the surface, the compressed air inside your body expands, causing pain and possibly rupture of tissues. It is for this reason that swimmers are urged to ascend slowly, which gives time for more gradual equalization of the pressure to occur, and to exhale as they ascend to the surface. This pertains to swimming pool depths as well as deeper dives.

SCUBA diving

The use of self-contained underwater breathing apparatus (SCUBA) introduces additional concerns because the swimmer can descend to much greater depths and stay there longer.

Because SCUBA diving presents unique physical forces and physiological responses which are not encountered in surface swimming or skin diving, people who take up this sport need formal instruction that includes detailed information on how to cope with its specific hazards.

Such instruction is offered by stores which sell the equipment, schools and colleges, YMCAs and YWCAs, swim clubs, etc.

We Live in a Gadget Culture

The idea of keeping physically fit is appealing, but many people are unwilling to do what it takes to achieve it. If we could package physical fitness and sell it, we would have many takers; people keep hoping that some mechanical gadget will offer an effortless means of achieving and maintaining physical fitness.

Although equipment cannot be substituted for physical effort, it can assist certain types of exercise. Here we will discuss some of the more commonly available types of exercise equipment and their relative merits.

Much of the fitness apparatus on the market is useful. Barbells and other free weights can be used to increase resistance to contracting muscles and thereby improve muscular strength, as was discussed in Chapter 5. Or you can use weight machines, the more expensive alternatives seen in many fitness centers, to achieve the same result.

Carrying weights by hand or around the wrists or ankles while jogging increases the effort involved, provided the runner steps as high, as far, and as fast as before. Joggers who decrease their pace or distance because of the added stress of the weights forfeit some or all of the potential benefit. Also, there is the possibility that weights may aggravate joint pain and other problems in the lower extremities. At any rate, research has not demonstrated the effectiveness of wearing such weights for improving either performance or $\dot{V}_{O_2}$ max.

Weighted belts, often in the form of lead-shot-filled pockets, are also available. Usually they are advertised as a way to increase fitness or maintain body weight. If you ascend a flight of stairs wearing such a belt, it is obvious that you do more work and place a greater load on your leg muscles. But as with the weights discussed above, we don't know whether people who wear these belts reduce their physical activity and therefore negate the possible benefits. A classic example of how the principle can be misunderstood involves a typist who sat at her desk all day wearing a weighted belt and smugly proclaimed the effortless weight loss that would soon be hers.

Stationary bicycles, treadmills, and rowing machines are useful for increasing and maintaining fitness. It is unlikely that the skeletal muscles or cardiovascular system recognize any difference between rowing out on the lake, and rowing a stationary machine at home or in a fitness center. The physiological effects are the same.

Indoor machines allow you to exercise regardless of the weather. Many people use stationary equipment effectively and happily in their ongoing fitness programs. Some watch TV or listen to music to add enjoyment. However, others find such exercise boring, so they quit doing it. (It is not uncommon to see classified ads in the newspaper for stationary bicycles which are "like new.") This is strictly a matter of individual preference.

A very inexpensive piece of equipment that can be used for aerobic activity is a jump rope. Rope skipping is a highly aerobic activity which ranks with jogging and fast cycling in rate of energy expenditure.

Watching television often is accused of having a negative effect on fitness; however, in some circumstances it can actually contribute to fitness. For example, if you have a video cassette player, you can use video tapes of aerobic dancing to help you exercise in the privacy and convenience of your own home.

Vibrating belts, on the other hand, involve passive activity. The energy required to resist the belt movement is very minimal, and therefore this equipment is not useful for maintaining fitness or body weight.

Some gadgets may possibly carry a medical risk. Electrical muscle stimulators are an example of this. Users of this apparatus attach electrodes to the skin over the muscles; repeated electrical charges cause contraction of the muscles. It is not known whether there might be some health hazards associated with the use of this equipment. Furthermore, the energy expended using this apparatus is minimal—just a little more than your resting metabolic rate. This is because only one small muscle group is stimulated, whereas when we walk, jog, run, or exercise in other ways, we use the large muscle groups of the back, legs, and arms.

New gagets are continually being developed for a gullible public. With the information in this chapter, you should be able to evaluate new items as they appear. Applying this knowledge and using common sense can help you cut through the marketing gimmicks, and determine which products are useful and which are designed simply to make money for the manufacturer.

The key fact to keep in mind is that flexibility, strength, and aerobic fitness are developed and maintained only through energy expenditure and the active use of muscles. Gadgets that claim to do the work for you generally don't produce fitness.

Dealing With Stress 7

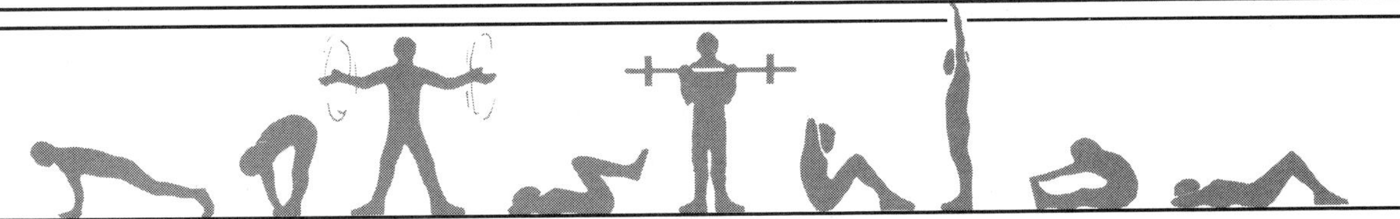

Outline

What makes you "up-tight"? An exam? Speaking in front of a group? Having somebody watch you play a sport that you're not very good at? Being around somebody you think is much more capable or affluent or attractive than you are? Thinking about your financial status?

Undoubtedly everybody has felt tense, nervous, or jittery in these or other situations; such feelings are indications of *psychological stress*. Although we have come to assume that a certain amount of such stress is an inevitable feature of contemporary life that people must learn to live with, we may sometimes become so stressed that it interferes with happy, healthy, productive living.

Fortunately, we can avoid becoming casualties of such stress: there are ways to manage stress so that it does not erode the quality of our lives.

In this chapter we will discuss how stress arises, how it can affect performance and health, and how you can relieve excessive stress by using various behavioral methods.

Stress—Who Needs It?

We're not saying that all stress is bad; it isn't. It can sometimes actually help a person improve his or her performance.

Consider stress in the lives of early humans: presumably, they encountered many situations in which they were physically threatened. Such stress was accompanied by physiological changes which quickly mobilized their bodily resources. For example, respiration and heart rate increased, blood pressure rose, and glycogen was converted to glucose and made available for quick energy. Such factors enabled people to perform at an extraordinary level—the classic "fight or flight" response. It sometimes made the difference as to whether or not they survived the danger.

Now if you are in a situation of physical danger—say that you are crossing the street and a car comes screeching around the corner toward you—you experience the same physiological reactions. You make a dash for the curb much faster than you ordinarily could. Without the sudden surge of energy that the stress produced in you, you could have been killed.

But in this day and age, physical threat is not the most frequent cause of our stress. More often, we produce our stress when we sense some sort of *nonphysical* "danger," such as an upcoming exam or job interview. Nonetheless, the same body changes that are associated with physical stress occur. In such cases *it is our thoughts*—not the circumstances themselves—*that create the stress* (Figure 7.1). Many situations

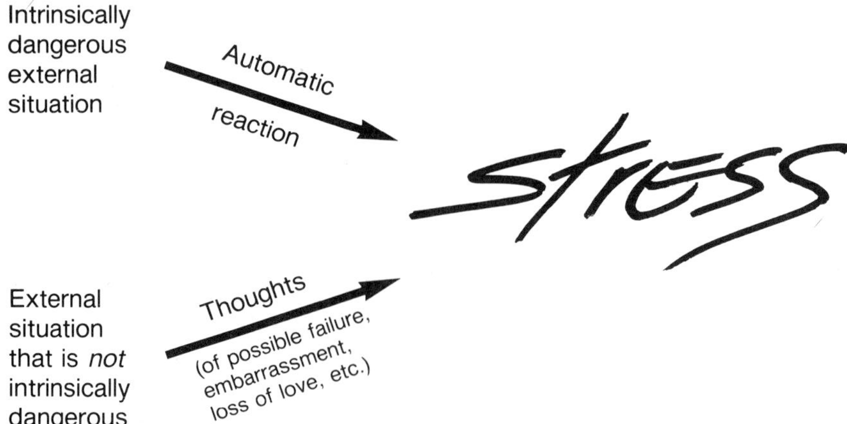

Figure 7.1   Origins of stress. Stress can be caused either by a situation that is physically dangerous, or from our perception that a situation carries risks of other kinds.

have elements of both; that is, there may be a small physical risk in a situation (such as airplane travel), but a person may grossly exaggerate the danger in his mind, creating much more stress than the amount of physical risk warrants.

In small amounts, even self-imposed stress can be beneficial. Probably you can think of instances in which you felt a little nervous about something you were about to do, but were able to channel that nervous energy into a better performance. Hans Selye, a noted researcher in the area of stress, referred to this as *eustress* (good stress). If we never felt any tension whatsoever, we might not accomplish much of anything.

But excessive stress creates *distress* (again as Selye used it) which can wreak havoc on mind and body. However, since most people use the word "stress" where Selye would have used "distress," we will continue to use the shortened term **stress** in this chapter. In the next section we will deal with the mental and physical effects of stress.

Stress: The unpleasant internal state which helps organisms prepare to cope with danger.

The Price of Too Much Stress

If we stress ourselves frequently, severely, and/or for prolonged periods, we may:

- Interfere with school, job, and social performance
- Increase the risk of cardiovascular diseases such as high blood pressure, migraine, and heart attack
- Increase the risk of ulcers
- Weaken the immune system
- Increase the likelihood of developing mental disorders

For these reasons, learning about stress and how to deal with it is an important part of any program that is designed to enhance overall health.

Let's begin by exploring the two major components of stress, the physical and the verbal. What do you notice about yourself when you are feeling stressed? If you were to list your reactions, you would find that they fall into two major categories—physical and verbal ("verbal" refers to what we think as well as what we say).

Physical aspects of stress

Physical symptoms reflect the adaptations your body makes to help you respond to an emergency, as we described earlier. Among the effects you may notice is muscle tension, especially in the face, neck, and back. You may be aware that your heart beats faster, your hands and feet get cold, your body shakes, your armpits are sweaty, your mouth is dry, your voice quavers, your stomach churns, and your head feels dizzy. Fortunately, most people do not have all of these symptoms at one time.

The physical aspects of stress vary from person to person. The assortment of physical symptoms you typically notice in yourself when you feel stressed may be quite different from those someone else may notice.

Verbal aspects of stress

What you think when you feel stressed is also important. You may size up a certain situation as difficult for you, and begin to make statements to yourself such as, "I know my parents will be upset with me if I don't do well on this exam," or "I'm afraid I'm going to fall flat on my face in front of everybody."

Such messages can cause the physiological features of stress to begin. When you feel such an effect and say something to yourself like, "I'm really getting weak in the knees. . . . Something really terrible must be wrong with me," the physiological reaction might be intensified. A positive feedback loop, a kind of vicious cycle, might be created (Figure 7.2).

Another way our words or thoughts can increase stress is when we expect a certain situation, person, or object to be stressful for us. Thinking such thoughts can make them so (a self-fulfilling prophecy). For example, if you expect an exam to be rugged, you are likely to intensify your stress—independent of the actual level of difficulty of the exam.

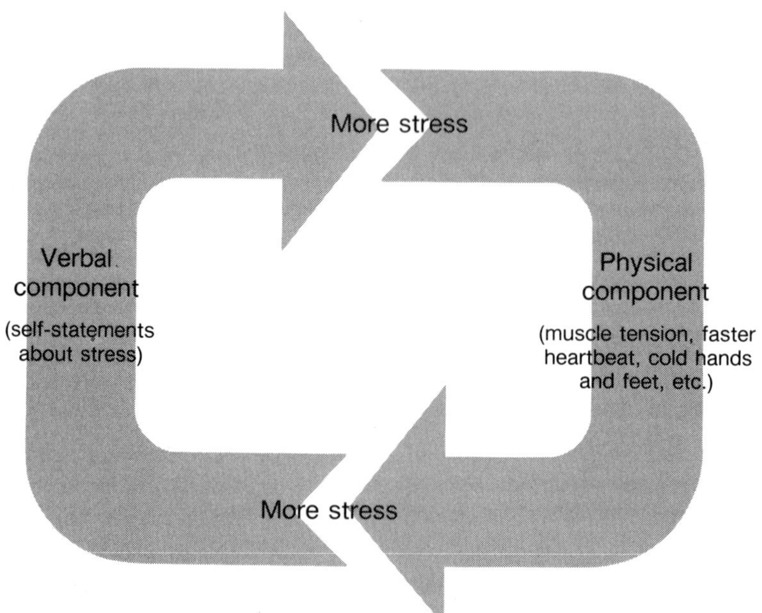

Figure 7.2 How physical and verbal factors interact to increase stress.

Since we create our own stress to some extent, situations that are stressful to one person are not necessarily stressful to another. However, mental-health workers have learned that there are certain life-events which are associated with some degree of stress for almost everybody.

What are these circumstances? Examples of events that are associated with stress in almost all of us are: experiencing the death of someone close to us, sexual difficulties, and getting in trouble with the police. These situations seem so obviously negative that we talk about them as though the events themselves provoked the stress (i.e., ''a stressful situation'').

What is less apparent is that some situations which at first glance seem positive can also cause stress. Such situations usually demand substantial change in our lives. Events such as marriage, promotion, and retirement are often stressful despite their apparently positive nature. It is helpful to know this; otherwise you may be surprised and upset with yourself for having mixed feelings about a situation in which everybody around you is saying, ''How wonderful! You must feel great!''

When several stressful circumstances are present at once, the stress is cumulative. The time around college graduation is often one of high stress because of the many important changes that are likely to occur at about the same time—such as leaving school, moving, and starting a new job.

Is it possible to measure the stress caused by various common life events? On the basis of extensive interviews and careful reviews of personal histories, Holmes and Rahe (1967) developed a list of common stressors and assigned points to each one corresponding to the amount of stress caused. The list is shown in Table 7.1. Note that seemingly positive events, such as marriage and retirement, are among the most stressful events. In subsequent research, it has been found that physical illness will often result if an individual has a high score.

The Holmes and Rahe scale certainly has its limitations. For one thing, some people won't find it useful because their concerns aren't represented: students, working mothers, and elderly could construct a different stress list more suitable to them. On the other hand, you might find the list useful as a way of anticipating and preparing for stressful events. In the next section, we will present some ways of managing the stress resulting from these events, as well as from those situations which are more individually stressful.

You Can Anticipate and Measure Stress

Fortunately, there are a number of methods a person can use for reducing stress. They involve interrupting the positive feedback loop described earlier and shown in Figure 7.2. Some people discover on their own an activity that works for them. For example, you may have found that doing crossword puzzles is very relaxing for you; somebody

Stress Management Procedures Can Help

Table 7.1 The Holmes-Rahe stress test

Event	Points
Death of spouse	100
Divorce	73
Marital separation	65
Jail term	63
Death of close family member	63
Personal injury or illness	53
Marriage	50
Fired at work	47
Marital reconciliation	45
Retirement	45
Change in health of family member	44
Pregnancy	40
Sex difficulties	39
Gain of new family member	39
Business readjustment	39
Change in financial state	38
Death of close friend	37
Change to different line of work	36
Change in number of arguments with spouse	35
Loan over $10,000	31
Foreclosure of mortgage or loan	30
Change in responsibilities at work	29
Son or daughter leaving home	29
Trouble with in-laws	29
Outstanding personal achievement	28
Spouse begins or stops work	26
Begin or end school	26
Change in living conditions	25
Revision of personal habits	24
Trouble with boss	23
Change in work hours or conditions	20
Change in residence	20
Change in schools	20
Change in recreation	19
Change in church activities	19
Change in social activities	18
Mortgage or loan less than $10,000	17
Change in sleeping habits	16
Change in number of family get-togethers	15
Change in eating habits	15
Vacation	13
Christmas	12
Minor violations of the law	11

else may unwind by reading or enjoying a favorite hobby. People with such activities may not need the techniques in this section; but for those who don't already have a healthy way of reducing stress, we offer the following four methods: aerobic exercise, relaxation training, systematic desensitization, and cognitive restructuring.

Aerobic exercise

Aerobic exercise can be used to reduce stress in both immediate and long-term ways. When a person does a single aerobic workout, he or she feels less tension for two to five hours afterward; psychologists refer to this short-term effect as a reduction in **state anxiety**, which is the anxiety you experience at any given time. Then, gradually, tension returns to pre-exercise levels. Knowing this may help people decide at what time during the day it would be best for them to work out.

There may also be a long-term, stress-reducing benefit of aerobic exercise: a person who exercises regularly may reduce his or her characteristic level of stress, or **trait anxiety**. A person who used to feel "uptight" at the slightest provocation may find that after exercising regularly for several weeks, he or she no longer becomes nervous as readily.

This benefit of exercise—that it reduces stress—is an example of *negative reinforcement*. That is, people exercise because an unpleasant internal state—stress—is reduced.

Aerobic exercise sometimes has been used to treat more serious psychological problems also. One study has shown that an exercise program was as effective in treating depression as was group therapy (Greist et al., 1979). However, this is not to say that a clinically or severely depressed person can substitute jogging for getting help from a psychologist or psychiatrist; professional help is in order for treating depression, but aerobic exercise may be a helpful part of a therapy program.

Can aerobic exercise go beyond reducing stress, and lift your spirits to higher-than-normal levels? Some people have suggested that running can elevate your mood, a phenomenon called the *"runner's high."* People describe the experience as a psychological lift they sometimes feel after they have been running for 35 or 40 minutes; they describe a euphoria, a heightened sense of well-being.

It has been theorized that running beyond a certain intensity and time may promote the release of endorphins, which are natural opiates (pain killers) produced within the body, and that these may be responsible for "runner's high." However, so far research has not established the prevalence of "runner's high" or the role of endorphins in producing it.

Relaxation training

Relaxation training is a procedure that helps people recognize tension in their muscles, and trains them to release that tension. Daily practice

State anxiety: Stress experienced at a particular time.

Trait anxiety: A person's general predisposition to become stressed.

Relaxation training: A method of reducing stress by recognizing and releasing muscle tension.

of the technique maintains the skill; then, whenever a person experiences muscular tension during the course of the day's activities, he or she can relax the affected muscles.

You can learn relaxation from a therapist in individual or group sessions, or possibly even from books (Davis, et al., 1980) or tapes. There is good evidence that if you learn to relax the voluntary muscles, you will reduce the other aspects of stress as well.

Certain conditions are important for learning and practicing relaxation. You will need a quiet room and comfortable furniture that completely supports your body, such as a bed, sofa, recliner, or overstuffed chair with a high-enough back to offer head support. Your clothes should be loose and comfortable. If you wear contact lenses, take them out.

Lie or sit in a way that allows you to feel as relaxed as possible, without tensing any muscles to hold your position; strategically-placed pillows may be helpful. Close your eyes. Then tense the muscles in an isolated region of your body enough so that you become familiar with the feeling of tension. The tension period should last 5 to 10 seconds. Produce only enough tension to become aware of what it feels like; don't overdo it. After 5 to 10 seconds, slowly release the tension, letting it go for about 45 to 60 seconds. Try to become aware of the feeling of decreasing tension as you relax. It is this feeling that you will use to reduce stress in the course of your daily activities.

You can work on relaxing small muscle groups, or you can focus on larger areas consisting of combined groups. The suggested sequence to use for relaxing muscles is as follows:

- Arms: dominant hand, forearm, and upper arm; nondominant hand, forearm, and upper arm
- Face: forehead, area around the eyes, mouth, and jaws
- Neck
- Torso: chest, shoulders, upper back, and stomach
- Legs: dominant thigh and calf; nondominant thigh and calf

Since you should concentrate on tensing and relaxing your muscles—and on how different those two conditions feel—you should not interrupt the process to think about what muscles to work on next. Therefore, it is helpful to have a record or tape that tells you the sequence.

Whatever degree of relaxation a person attains at the first attempt, he or she usually is increasingly successful with further practice. For maximal benefit, practice the technique twice each day in 15- to 20-minute sessions with at least three hours between them. Select a time of day when you do not feel rushed; you can't hurry relaxation.

A book that teaches one variation of relaxation training is *The Relaxation Response* by Herbert Benson (1975). Benson's method makes use of some features of relaxation training as described above, and also borrows from transcendental meditation (TM), a practice that has its roots in Eastern philosophy. On the surface, a method that blends a traditional method with one that is derived from philosophy may seem unacceptable to the behavioral scientist. However, Benson has used scientific methods to study and modify certain features of TM, and, having found them useful, incorporated them into his stress-reduction technique minus their mystical overtones.

Systematic desensitization

Systematic desensitization is a method for reducing stress that involves gradual exposure, via the imagination, to a stress-producing situation while a person is very relaxed. If the relaxation can be maintained in the imaginary situation, it may be possible to transfer it to the real situation.

Systematic desensitization: A procedure to reduce stress by imagining increasingly disturbing situations while relaxed.

We can use fear of public speaking as an example: Let's say that you want to get rid of the rapid heartbeat, dry mouth, cold feet, and shaking hands that you experience when you make a presentation to a group.

Before you begin systematic desensitization, use your past experience to rank stressful speaking situations: that is, make a list from the most stressful situation to the least stressful. Your list might include items such as these, although this is not an exhaustive list:

1. Speaking to a large group of hostile strangers in an unfamiliar setting on a difficult, controversial topic
2. Speaking to a large group of strangers on a familiar, noncontroversial topic
3. Speaking to a small group of strangers on a familiar, noncontroversial topic
4. Speaking to a small group of friendly people on a familiar, noncontroversial topic
5. Conversing with a small group of friendly people on a mutually enjoyable topic

Then, with your list in front of you, get yourself into a relaxed state by applying what you learned in the section on relaxation training.

Next, imagine that you are in the situation at the bottom of your list, the one that evokes the least anxiety. When you can imagine that situation without becoming anxious, or when you can dissipate any anxiety that you feel, move on to imagining the next situation. Work your way up the list in this manner until you can imagine the most stressful situation either without becoming anxious or with the ability to reduce anxiety by means of relaxation. The payoff will come when you find that you can cope with the actual situations without becoming anxious.

This technique of systematic desensitization is a more comfortable way to overcome fears than the methods proposed by certain folk advice. For example, if you are thrown from a horse (literally or figuratively), you now know that you do not need to immediately remount the beast as the only way to overcome your fear. Or if you want to learn to swim but are afraid of deep water, isn't it good to know that there is a less traumatic way to reach your goal than to be thrown in over your head?

Cognitive restructuring

It is also possible to reduce stress by dealing directly with the thoughts that give rise to it; **cognitive restructuring** is a technique that can help accomplish this. To use this technique you must become aware of the self-statements that result in feelings such as anxiety, fear, depression, or anger.

As you think back to a situation that had a strong negative emotional charge for you, it isn't easy to recall the various thoughts you had at the time. However, it is useful to uncover them, because you can bring about changes in the feelings by identifying and modifying the thoughts that initiated them.

To become aware of the thoughts involved, it can be helpful to keep a diary of your thoughts, as shown in Self-check 7.1. Each time you feel anxious about something, write down what you are thinking about and how you feel at the time. Figure 7.3 gives an example of a completed diary for part of one day.

After you have made entries for several days, review your diary to see whether you are producing unnecessary stress by thinking types of thoughts that are counterproductive to your emotional well-being. The following paragraphs describe some common types of negative thinking.

One type of counterproductive thinking is **filtering**, in which a person concentrates on the negative aspects of a situation. For example, think of a student looking over an assignment that earned a grade of B+; the instructor has written many positive comments on the paper along with a few negative ones. If the person were filtering, he would quickly bypass the positive messages and focus on the negatives: "Look at that. I messed up two of the references. What dumb mistakes—I just copied them wrong. The professor must think I'm really careless. Well, I guess I am. With that kind of sloppiness, I probably didn't even deserve the B+."

If you think you are prone to this type of thinking, try to stand back from the situation and see it as a whole, allowing yourself credit for its positive aspects. You can reduce your stress by keeping the negatives in perspective.

Another pitfall can be **polarized thinking**, in which you view yourself or your world in an "all-or-nothing" light. You see a situation as either all good or all bad. You are either a complete success or an abject failure; either brilliant or totally stupid; a suave sophisticate, or an absolute clod. You cannot see the possibility of being in between.

Cogniture restructuring: A procedure to reduce stress by changing the thoughts that give rise to it.

Filtering: Focusing on negative aspects of a situation while ignoring its positive features.

Polarized thinking: Viewing the world as black and white, rather than in shades of gray.

Self-check 7.1   A thoughts diary

An essential part of cognitive restructuring is to discover what you are thinking when you experience stress. You can use this form to determine your stress-producing thoughts.

Time	Situation	Thoughts	Feelings

Figure 7.3   An example of how a thoughts diary (Self-check 7.1) might look.

An essential part of cognitive restructuring is to discover what you are thinking when you experience stress. You can use this form to determine your stress-producing thoughts.

Time	Situation	Thoughts	Feelings
8:20 AM	Can't understand lecture.	Everybody else looks like they get it. I must be stupid.	depression
10:00 AM	Person next to me in Economics is almost done with his term paper.	He's way ahead of me. I'll never finish mine on time.	anxiety
11:45 AM	Was supposed to meet Sara at Union at 11:30.	She'll be annoyed that I'm late. I don't judge my time very well.	anxiety
1:00 PM	Made comment in discussion section. TA says I sound like I know the material.	Other students look like they think I'm showing off.	depression
5:00 PM	Haven't had time to get birthday card for Mom.	She'll feel hurt if it's late. She'll think I don't care.	anxiety
7:30 PM	Working in the library; given a lot of books to shelve.	I'll have to work late. This job takes more time than I thought.	anger

Polarized thinking can create considerable stress for two reasons. First, being either the absolute best or worst are intrinsically stressful situations; second, this image probably does not square with reality. If you imagine that you are at the top of the heap in some regard, you are bound to be disappointed eventually. The belief that you are "dead last" is probably also wrong, and it may discourage you from trying to improve.

The way out of this sort of thinking is to realize that few people or situations are black or white; most are shades of gray. People and situations are not usually absolutely good or bad, but rather are located on a continuum, and are able to shift along it.

A related type of counterproductive thinking is called **catastrophizing**. In this case, when a person thinks ahead to an upcoming situation, he or she anticipates the worst possible outcome. Before an exam, such a person might think, "What if my mind goes blank when the exam starts? If I flunk this exam, I'm likely to get a D in the course. With a grade like that, I'll get kicked out of my major, and there go my hopes for a career in hospital administration, and that's the only thing I want to do."

The antidote for this is to imagine the other possible scenarios as well. Realize that you'll probably be well prepared for some parts of the exam, and not so well prepared for others. Instead of worrying, it would be more productive to invest your time in one last review of the course material.

Finally, having unrealistically high, inflexible expectations of yourself can create stress. People who have a large catalogue of "shoulds," "oughts," and "musts" that they try to live by may be burdening themselves with impossible goals.

Besides, how many perfect people do you know? If you know some (or can imagine them), do you find them likeable? Chances are, you have discovered that some of the characteristics that make people interesting and appealing are their unique imperfections. The Chinese include an intentional deviation from the pattern in their beautiful rugs to make them one-of-a-kind and therefore of greater worth. Perhaps we should value our own minor imperfections in a similar light. People who continually criticize themselves for falling short of the highest mark—which may be unattainable anyway—would reduce their stress if they devoted less mind-time to such negative thinking.

A good description of cognitive restructuring is contained in the book *Thoughts and Feelings: The Art of Cognitive Stress Intervention* by McKay, Davis and Fanning.

Biofeedback

Because so much attention has been given to it in the popular press, you have probably already heard of **biofeedback**; this is why we include it here. It is less likely to be used by the average person than the methods above, though, because it requires sophisticated equip-

Catastrophizing: Focusing on the worst-case scenario when thinking about an upcoming event.

Biofeedback: A stress management procedure in which information about some physiological aspect of stress is presented and used to reduce stress.

ment and professional expertise, making it too impractical and expensive for ordinary use. However, if you were using biofeedback to reduce stress, you would receive and act on information about the physical aspects of your stress reaction. You would use equipment that would monitor your heart rate, muscle tension, or some other physical stress reaction. The equipment would also give you feedback regarding your reaction and you would use this information to change the reaction. For example, if you were hooked up to a machine that monitored muscle tension in your forehead, you might hear a signal such as a clicking noise, that would be correlated with the amount of tension; the more rapid the clicks, the higher the tension. You would try to slow down the clicks and hence relax your forehead. Once you learned this, you would try to apply this skill to relieve tension when you are not connected to the machine.

Other methods of stress reduction

The methods described above represent the major types of stress-reduction techniques currently recognized as effective by behavioral psychologists. You may also encounter techniques with other names. Some may be modifications of the methods described in this chapter. Others may be based on unproven theories about how to reduce stress or, at worst, may be complete scams to take your money. Therefore, before you commit yourself to any method, consider whether it uses a technique known to be effective, and whether it is worth its price.

Although the techniques discussed in this chapter are suitable for use by the general public, people who are under very severe stress may have difficulty applying them successfully. If this is your case, a mental health professional can help you select an appropriate technique and guide you in its use.

In addition, before you try to use one of the procedures described, it will probably be helpful for you to read about it in one of the references listed in the source notes at the back of this book.

Virtually everybody, at some time of life, experiences levels of stress that interfere with happy, healthy, productive living. It is not necessary to put up with such a burden: many people can manage their own stress successfully with the methods outlined in this chapter.

Nutrition Basics: Food Becomes You 8

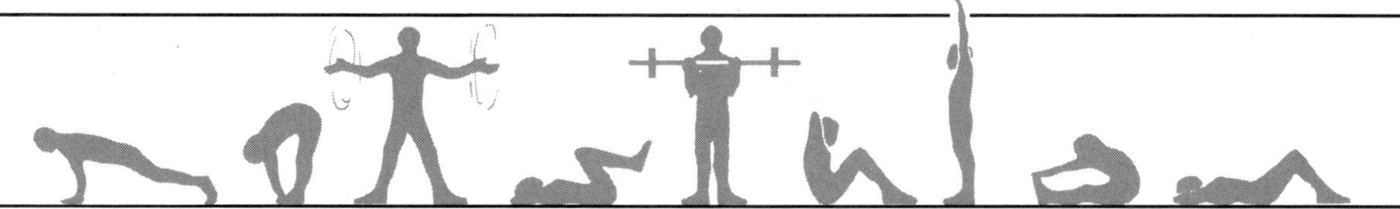

Outline

So you want to know what you should eat to be healthy. You may be thinking, "Let's get right to the bottom line. Just give me a diet that will make me feel great, perform well, and look good . . . and then keep me that way."

Unfortunately, it's not that simple. For one thing, we can't promise you all of that from any diet; those expectations are out of line with what good nutrition can produce all by itself. Although good nutrition certainly contributes to a sense of well-being, top performance, and appearance, it is only one lifestyle factor among the many that influence your fitness. You have already learned that exercise and relief of stress play important roles in good health as well. Good nutrition can't substitute for exercise or a healthy state of mind, but it can work together with those factors and others toward your total health.

For another thing, the "right diet" is a somewhat individual matter. Although all people need the same nutrients for growth, reproduction, and maintenance of health, the *amount* of a particular nutrient one person needs is likely to differ from what another person requires, since nutritional needs vary according to body size, sex, reproductive status (whether a woman is or is not pregnant or lactating), activity level, age, and other individual factors. Therefore there is no such thing as one diet that is right for everybody.

Another reason we can't give you a preplanned diet is that the diet might contain some foods you don't like and wouldn't eat; or it might omit some of your favorite foods, which would be just as unacceptable. Of course you want to eat foods that you like, and we cannot know what you prefer.

Therefore the thrust of the nutrition chapters will be to give you tools to use for understanding, evaluating, and planning your own diet. The goal is to help you be as healthy as nutrition can make you.

In this chapter, we will give you some basic background information about nutrients and why you need them.

Nutrients Do Three Things

Nutrients have three functions in your body: (1) they are the building materials for body structures, (2) they provide energy, and (3) they serve as regulators of body processes.

Contribute to body structure

The expressions "Food becomes you" and "You are what you eat" speak the truth: your body is composed of nutrients that you—or your mother when she was pregnant with you—consumed and biochemically reconstructed into the stuff of which you are made.

This is not to say that you can completely determine what you become by what you eat. Your body's physical potential is limited by your genetic background; but the degree to which you achieve that potential is influenced substantially by nutrition. For example, your genes (the cellular components that determine hereditary characteristics) contain instructions for developing a certain amount and distribution of muscle tissue. Eating more meat cannot add bulk to your biceps; but exercise plus a good diet allows you to develop your muscle mass up to your inborn potential.

Provide fuel

Another vital function of nutrients is to provide energy. Without energy, life ceases.

Energy, as we indicated earlier, is measured in kcalories. Most adults use between 1500 and 3500 kcalories in a day, depending on body size, how muscular they are, and their physical activity level.

Regulate processes

The third important function that nutrients perform is the regulation of body processes. The metabolic reactions that take place in your body do not occur in random fashion; they are intricately controlled. Many nutrients are involved in your finely tuned system of biochemical checks and balances.

Essential Nutrients

Humans require close to 50 specific substances that must be taken into the body preformed and in sufficient quantities to meet the body's needs for growth, reproduction, and maintenance of health; these are called **nutrients**. The nutrients are distinguished from thousands of nonessential substances that we consume in food in that the nonessentials either can be produced within the body or are not needed by it.

The nutrients are grouped into six classes: *water, carbohydrates, lipids* (commonly called fats), *proteins, vitamins,* and *minerals.*

The classes of nutrients needed in the largest amounts are water, carbohydrates, lipids, and proteins; for this reason they are called *macronutrients.* Vitamins and minerals, which are needed in very small amounts, are called *micronutrients.*

Scientists have determined what level people need for many nutrients, and the results are published in the document called *Recommended Dietary Allowances* (the RDA or RDAs), which are revised at approximately five-year intervals. The RDAs represent goals for people in the United States: people who get 70 to 100 percent of the levels of nutrients suggested by the RDAs are considered to have acceptable intakes.

Look ahead for a moment to the RDA table in the next chapter on page 168 (Table 9.4); note that there are separate recommendations for different population groups, according to age, sex, and reproductive status. We will use the RDAs in Chapter 9 to help evaluate your diet.

Some people believe that the more we get of the essential nutrients, the better off we'll be. This is not true: more is not always better. In fact, there is risk from getting too much; Figure 8.1 makes the point that *serious problems can result from either inadequate OR excessive intake of nutrients.*

People who experience harm from nutrient overdose are usually people who have used concentrated nutritional supplements inappropriately. Some people take many times the recommended levels and thereby put themselves at risk of **toxicity**. There is much we don't know about excessive nutrient intake, because such studies are unethical to do on humans; therefore people who take high levels of nutrients experiment on themselves.

The best way to get the levels of nutrients you need is *to consume the right kinds and amounts of foods.* Generally speaking, supplements

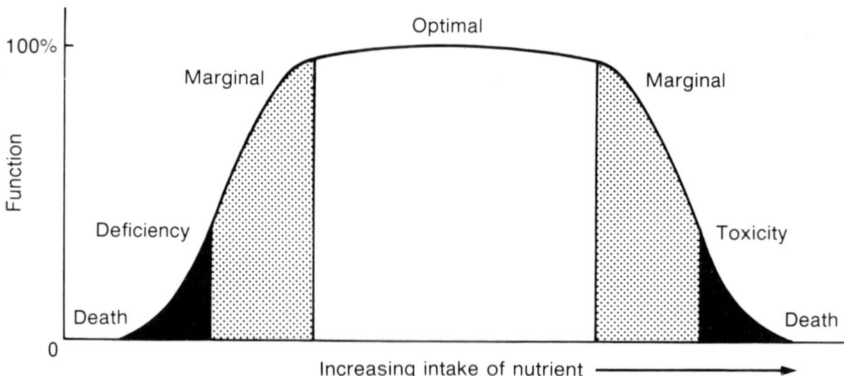

Figure 8.1   The effects of various levels of nutrient intake. Either extreme—too little or too much of a nutrient—can have disastrous effects on growth, reproduction, and health.

are a second-best source of nutrients. However, in certain circumstances—such as pregnancy, lactation, or illness—moderate levels of supplements are useful. We will discuss who might benefit from supplements in Chapter 10.

While remembering the advice given above, let's move on to more information about the six categories of essential nutrients.

Water: too vital to take for granted

In a way, you could make a case for water being the "most essential" nutrient, since without water you would die in only a few days, whereas you could last a lot longer without other essential nutrients. You get a sense of why water is so important when you know how much of the body is composed of water; it accounts for 50 to 60 percent of the typical adult's body weight.

All tissues contain water. Certainly, body fluids such as blood, saliva, and tears are largely water. But even very hard materials contain water: over one-fourth of the weight of bone is water. Water provides the environment in which the body's biochemical reactions happen; it transports materials into, through, and out of the body; it lubricates the body; and it helps regulate its temperature.

The health of all body systems depends on their adequate hydration. As we saw in Chapter 6, if you lose as little as 3 percent of your body weight as water, your physical performance begins to suffer. With greater losses, physical and mental stress and loss of function become more severe; at approximately 12 percent of weight loss as water, your circulatory system will collapse, resulting in death.

To keep the body properly hydrated, fluid that leaves the body must be replaced with an equal intake of water (Figure 8.2). The typical adult loses between two and three quarts of water each day via urine, skin, respiration, and feces (solid waste). Normally, we replace the majority of that by drinking beverages in response to our thirst, but we can also

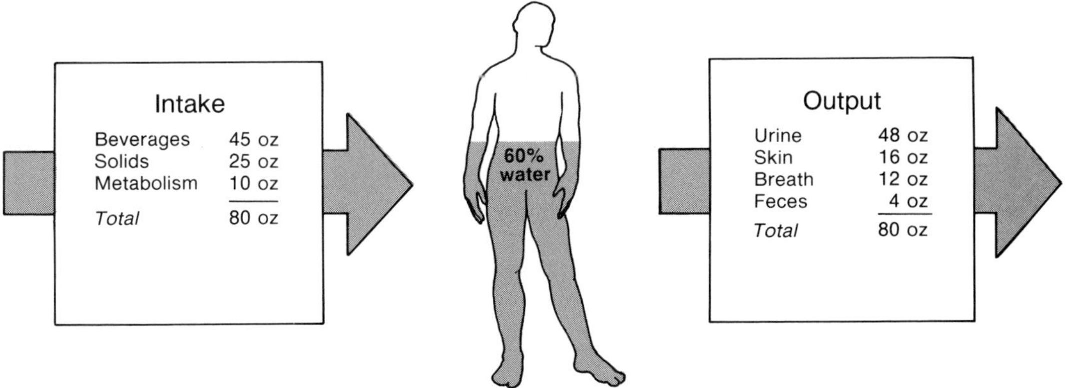

Figure 8.2 Maintaining water balance. Body water losses must be replaced to keep all systems functioning optimally; average daily adult output and intake are 2 to 3 quarts (64–96 ounces). This figure shows typical distribution of intake and output, but there is much individual variation.

get variable amounts of water from foods, some of which are over 90 percent water (e.g., fresh fruits and vegetables). In addition, a small amount of water is produced in the body from biochemical processes.

Although normally thirst can guide your water replacement quite effectively, there are a few situations in which thirst is not an adequate indicator of how much water you need. When you are sick, or when you are perspiring heavily from activity, you generally need more water than the amount that your thirst prompts you to drink. For example, a person who plays a vigorous tennis match on a very warm day and then sits in the sun to watch the next game may lose two to three times as much water on that day as our average values suggest, but may not get sufficiently thirsty to totally compensate for this loss on the day it occurred.

Water needs are influenced by several different factors, such as body size, how much you perspire in response to air temperature and physical activity, your clothing, and whether you have consumed any substances that promote fluid loss, such as alcohol or caffeine.

Carbohydrates: fine for fuel

Sugars, dextrins, and *starches* all belong to the carbohydrate family. Sugars are sweet, soluble, and simple in their chemical structure; major sources are fruits and vegetables, milk, and foods to which cane sugar, beet sugar, honey, or syrups have been added. Dextrins and starches are not as sweet or as soluble and are structurally more complex, which is why they are often referred to as "complex carbohydrates." Vegetables, grains, nuts, and seeds are their major dietary sources.

Of the three functions that nutrients have, carbohydrates serve primarily as energy providers. It is typical for our body cells to produce about half of our energy from carbohydrates and the other half from lipids, with a much smaller amount coming from proteins. But because the amount of carbohydrate in the body is so much smaller than the fat reserves, we need to restock it frequently by consuming generous amounts of carbohydrates. We should take in at least half—50 to 60 percent—of our kcalories from carbohydrates in the diet. Some of this carbohydrate will be used fairly quickly for energy; some carbohydrate will be stored as glycogen; and any remainder will be converted to body fat.

Carbohydrates provide 4 kcalories per gram. (A gram is about 1/30 of an ounce.) Therefore, a teaspoon of table sugar, which weighs 4 to 5 grams, provides approximately 20 kcalories. Another example: a slice of bread contains about 1 gram of sugar and 12 grams of starch; together, the 13 grams of carbohydrate provide 52 kcalories. (A slice of bread usually contains about 80 kcalories; the other kcalories come from the small amounts of fat and protein that are also present.) Figure 8.3 shows the carbohydrate content of various foods. Notice that foods often contain more than one type of carbohydrate: a carrot, for example, contains both sugar and starch.

Carbohydrates occur in some foods in which you may not expect them, such as commercially prepared soups, luncheon meats, and coffee whiteners. You can identify carbohydrates that have been added to some foods by reading the lists of ingredients on food labels. Here are some carbohydrates commonly added to foods:

- *Sugars*: glucose, dextrose, fructose, levulose, lactose, maltose, sucrose (the chemical names of most sugars have an -ose ending), honey, corn syrup, corn syrup solids, turbinado sugar, brown sugar, total invert sugar
- *Sugar alcohols*, which are closely related to sugars: sorbitol, mannitol
- *Dextrins* and *starches*: dextrin, corn starch, wheat starch, hydrolyzed starch, modified starch, malted grains

Figure 8.4 shows an example of an ingredient label. You can get a rough idea of how much of each ingredient is present from the order in which they are listed: the ingredient that weighs the most is listed first, the one that weighs the least is listed last.

Most normally healthy adults consume between 200 and 400 grams of carbohydrate in a day. However, many Americans consume less than half of their energy as carbohydrate, and should take in more carbohydrate than they do.

Be aware, though, that all carbohydrate-containing foods are not of the same overall nutritional value. Foods that have a substantial amount of added sugar are of lower nutritional quality than items without added sugar, because concentrated sugar adds little or nothing but kcalories. It is nutritionally advantageous to eat fewer highly sugared

Figure 8.3 Kinds and amounts of carbohydrates in some foods.

Food	Amount	Carbohydrates (grams)
Fruits and vegetables		
Fruit or fruit juice (no added sugar)	½ cup	
Fruit (in heavy syrup)	½ cup	
Potatoes, corn, peas	½ cup	
Carrots, beets	½ cup	
Leafy greens, broccoli	1 cup	
Grain products		
White bread	1 slice	
Whole grain bread	1 slice	
Corn flakes	1 ounce	
Bran cereal	1 ounce	
Pasta or rice	½ cup	
Bagel	½	
Plain oatmeal cookies	2 medium	
Dairy products		
Milk (no milk solids added)	1 cup	
Milk (milk solids added)	1 cup	
Plain yogurt (with solids)	1 cup	
Sweetened fruit yogurt (with milk solids)	1 cup	
Ice cream	1½ cup	
Hard cheese	1⅓ ounce	
Meats and alternates		
Meat, fish, poultry	2 ounces	
Eggs	2	
Nuts	½ cup	
Legumes (starchy beans and peas)	1 cup	
Others		
Sugar, honey, molasses, etc.	1 tablespoon	
Jelly, jam	1 tablespoon	
Gelatin dessert	½ cup	
Cola beverage	12 ounce can	
Cherry pie (2 crust)	1/7 of 7-inch pie	

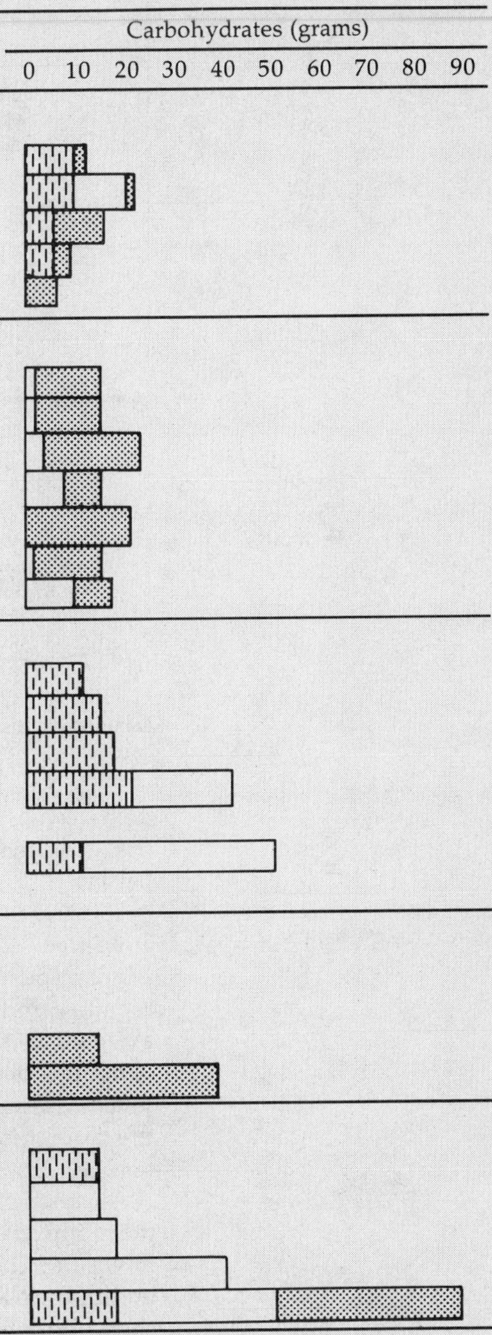

Carbohydrates (grams) scale: 0 10 20 30 40 50 60 70 80 90

Key: Naturally occurring sugars; added sugars; starches and dextrins.

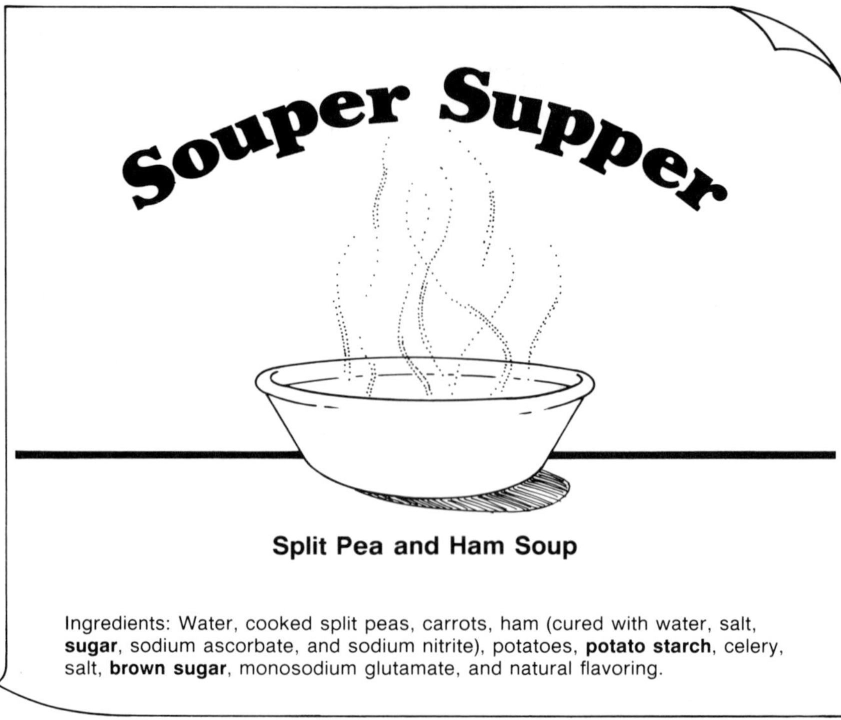

Ingredients: Water, cooked split peas, carrots, ham (cured with water, salt, **sugar**, sodium ascorbate, and sodium nitrite), potatoes, **potato starch**, celery, salt, **brown sugar**, monosodium glutamate, and natural flavoring.

Figure 8.4   Carbohydrates in a list of ingredients on a label. Various forms of carbohydrates are commonly added to processed foods to change their taste, consistency, or texture. Added carbohydrates are shown in boldface type.

foods while increasing your intake of starchy foods and unsugared fruits, which provide vitamins, minerals, and other nutrients in the bargain.

Fiber: Carbohydrate that cannot be digested by humans.

There is also another type of carbohydrate called **fiber** that deserves attention. We are discussing it separately because it is not a major energy source like sugars, starches, and dextrins. In the main, fiber remains undigested as it moves through the digestive tract and it is excreted in the feces (solid waste) intact. Even this passive role is of benefit, though; the presence of bulk due to fiber in the intestine gives your intestinal muscles exercise as they move fecal material through the tract. Since it is axiomatic that muscles need to do work to stay healthy, fiber contributes to intestinal health.

Another effect of fiber in the diet is that it causes fecal material to move through the intestinal tract more quickly than material that is lower in fiber; therefore, it decreases the likelihood of constipation. In addition, there is some evidence that it reduces the risk of cancer of the large intestine, although this has not been proved conclusively.

Although the amount of fiber in the average American diet is lower than most fiber researchers think it should be, it is quite possible for most people to get the right amount by eating foods that naturally contain it. The cell walls of all plant foods are made of fiber, with particularly large amounts in the outer (bran) layers of grains and in the peels and seeds of fruits and vegetables. Therefore, by eating at least two servings of whole grain products each day (such as brown rice, oatmeal, or whole wheat cereals and breads) and at least four servings of fruit and vegetable each day (such as unpeeled apples, corn, kidney beans, spinach, broccoli, or raspberries) you will get adequate fiber. People who do not eat items that are naturally high in fiber can get their fiber by eating a serving of high-fiber cereal or adding 2 to 3 tablespoons of refined bran to the diet per day. However, you should not consume much more, because in larger amounts, fiber may interfere with the body's ability to use certain necessary minerals.

There is another type of fiber—*soluble fiber*—which functions differently in the body than the *insoluble fiber* just discussed. Soluble fiber is extracted from certain plants and added to foods in small amounts to achieve a desired thickness or texture, or to give the product stability. Pectin, agar, carrageenan, locust bean gum, xanthan gum, and alginates are examples of such high-fiber additives: but do not count on such additives to provide the benefits mentioned earlier for insoluble fiber because the amount of fiber you get from these additives is very small and their activity is not the same.

Lipids: a mixed blessing

Lipids, or fats, perform many different functions in the body; in fact, lipids play structural, energy-providing, and regulating roles. The most familiar form of lipid in the body is in **adipose tissue**, which includes the layer of fat under the skin. This layer is an effective insulator of the body. Other adipose tissue acts as shock absorbers: approximately half your body fat is found in pads that cushion your internal organs.

Adipose tissue: Collectively, cells that specialize in the storage of fat in the body.

There are other beneficial roles that lipids play. Lipids in food (both fats and oils are lipids) promote the absorption of fat-soluble vitamins in the digestive tract. In addition, lipids are the stuff of which some hormones are made. (Hormones, such as epinephrine and estrogen, are chemical messengers that affect many body functions including metabolism and reproductive capacity.) Lipids are an important part of the membranes that surround every body cell, and also form a protective covering for nerve cells. One form of lipid is converted to a vitamin, and other lipids are components of secretions produced by the body to aid in digestion. Yet another form of lipid, called *linoleic acid*, is regarded as essential because people whose diets are devoid of it for a number of months develop a serious rash and fail to thrive.

You already know another important function of lipids: they are a major source of energy. They are a more concentrated source than carbohydrates, since lipids yield 9 kcalories per gram and carbohydrates yield only 4 kcalories per gram. Normally, people take in between 50 and 150 grams of lipids per day.

Even though lipids serve many important functions, there are negative effects of overconsumption. Excessive intake is related to obesity and also to increased risk of cardiovascular disease and cancer. To reduce such risks, most people should limit their intake of fat to no more than 30 percent of total kcalories. Since the average American intake is approximately 40 percent, many of us would be better off to decrease our intake of fat. The next chapter will show you how to calculate what percentage of your kcaloric intake comes from fat, carbohydrate, and protein.

Lipids are prevalent in the American diet, since they are naturally present in both foods of animal origin (e.g., meats, eggs, and milk) and in plant foods (e.g., nuts, seeds, and avocadoes). Other foods are high in fat because substantial amounts of fat or oils have been used in making them. For example, butter is often used as an ingredient in cookies, and oil is a component of many salad dressings. More than half of the fat we consume is likely to be hidden in our food in such ways. Table 8.1 shows the amount of lipids in various foods.

There is another issue that is important besides the quantitative one, and that is the *type* of fat that is consumed. Fats can be categorized, based on their chemical structures, as glycerides (mono-, di-, or triglycerides); phospholipids; or sterols. Furthermore, glycerides can be either saturated, monounsaturated, polyunsaturated, or hydrogenated. Rather than explaining those terms here, we will save that discussion for the chapter on cardiovascular disease, Chapter 9, because the terms have special significance there.

Nonetheless, at this point you should recognize that those terms are descriptors for lipids; you will see some of them used on nutrition labels. Some lipids such as monoglycerides, diglycerides, and lecithin (a phospholipid) are usually just used in small amounts as processing additives, and do not add much to the lipid content of food. Figure 8.5 shows an example of a nutrition label that includes several different lipids.

Proteins: the stuff of life

For thousands of years, people have understood that protein was important in the diet: the Greeks coined our word for it from their word *protos*, which means *first*. In fact, there is some protein in everything that lives. Living systems of all kinds need it in order to grow, reproduce, and repair and maintain themselves. There's no doubt that protein is essential.

Another way of demonstrating its importance is to point out that protein performs all of the basic functions of nutrients. It is a structural component of every cell in the body. Protein also acts as a regulator in many ways because it is the substrate from which several important biochemical materials are made: *enzymes* (which regulate the rate of biochemical reactions), *antibodies* (which help defend you from infec-

Table 8.1   Amounts of lipids in various foods

Lipid (gm)	Fruits and vegetables	Grain products	Milk and milk products	Meats and alternates	Combination foods	Limited extras
35				Walnuts (2 oz)		
30				Peanuts roasted in oil (2 oz) Dry roasted peanuts (2 oz)	Pecan pie (⅐ of pie)	
25						
20	Avocado (½)		Ice cream (½ c)		Chicken and noodles (1 c)	Italian salad dressing (1 oz)
15		{ Fried snack foods (1 oz) Frosted chocolate cake (2 oz) Oatmeal cookies (3 small)	Processed cheese (2 oz) Cheddar cheese (1⅓ oz)	Bologna (2 oz) { Fried fish, chicken (2 oz) Ham, ground beef (2 oz) Eggs (2)	Fruit pie (⅙ of pie) Lasagna (12 oz)	{ Cream cheese (1⅓ oz) French salad dressing (1 oz)
10	Potato chips (1 oz)		Whole milk (1 c)			Bacon (2 slices) { Oil, butter, margarine, mayonnaise (1 t) Sour cream (2 T)
5		Quick breads (1 slice) Plain bread (1 slice)	2% milk (1 c)	Broiled chicken, no skin (2 oz)	Pizza (¼ of 12″ cheese pie) Vegetable beef soup (1 c)	
0	Most plain fresh, frozen, canned fruits and vegetables (½ c)	Plain rice, pasta, most cereal (½ c)	Skim milk (1 c)	Cooked legumes (1 c)		

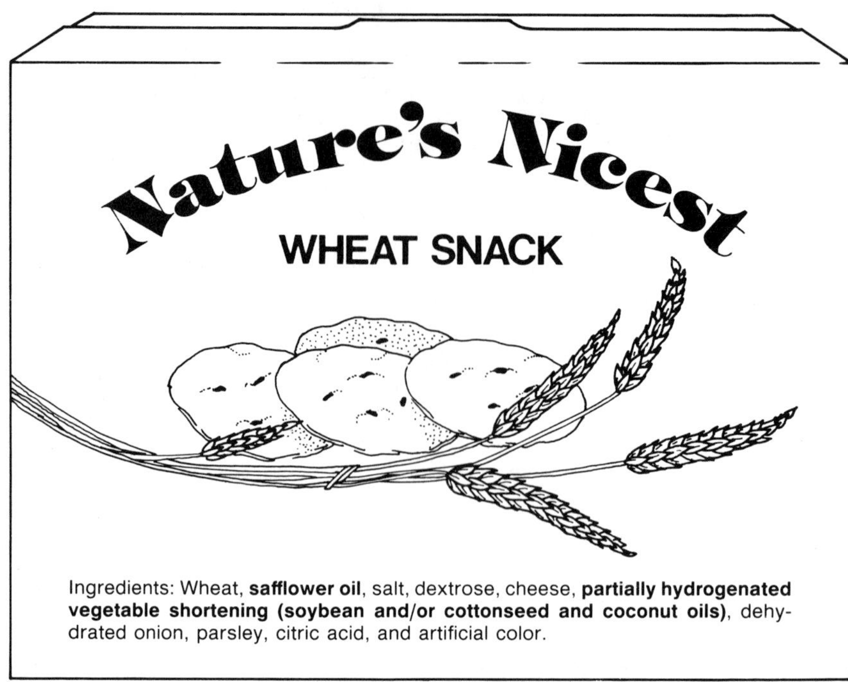

Figure 8.5 Lipids in a list of ingredients on a label. Lipids are commonly used as ingredients in processed foods; they add flavor, consistency and satiety value (hunger satisfaction). Added lipids are shown in boldface type.

tion), and some *hormones* are made of protein. It also helps regulate body fluid levels and the body's acidity and alkalinity.

Finally, protein has energy potential. Although only a small proportion of the energy you use in a day usually comes from protein, larger amounts can be metabolized if you have not consumed enough carbohydrate and fat to meet most of your energy needs. Protein, like carbohydrate, furnishes approximately 4 kcalories per gram.

Most foods as found in nature contain at least some protein. Those that contain the most protein are animal muscle tissues (e.g., meat, poultry, fish); eggs; milk and its products; starchy beans and peas (categorically called legumes); and some nuts. Other vegetables and grains contain smaller amounts. Highly refined foods (sugars and sweets, fats and oils, and alcoholic beverages) contain virtually no protein. Table 8.2 gives amounts typically present in average servings of various foods.

Overall, from 10 to 15 percent of the kcalories in your diet should come from protein. The average American gets almost double the amount he or she needs, so it is tempting to say that nobody needs to worry about protein intake. However, since there can be large deviations from the average, it is worthwhile to check your intake and needs. The next chapter will describe two ways to do this.

Table 8.2 Amounts of protein in various foods

Protein (gm)	Fruits and vegetables	Grain products	Milk and milk products	Meats and alternates	Combination foods	Limited extras
20				Lean chicken (2 oz)		
15				Peanuts (½ c) Lean beef (2 oz) Peanut butter (¼ c) Fish (2 oz) Tofu (6 oz) Eggs (2)		
			Processed cheese (2 oz)		Bean burrito (6 oz) Spaghetti & meatballs (1 c) 12″ cheese pizza (¼ pie)	
10			Hard cheese (1⅓ oz) Ice cream (1½ c) Milk (1 c) Pudding (1 c)		Macaroni and cheese (1 c) Chicken chow mein (1 c)	
5	Peas (½ c) Corn, potatoes (½ c)	Popcorn (3 c) Bread roll (1) Pasta, cereal (½ c) Tortilla, waffle (1) Cookies (3 small)			Cream of mushroom soup (1 c) Vegetable beef soup (1 c)	Gelatin dessert (½ c) Cream cheese (1½ oz)
0	Fruit—all kinds (½ c) Lettuce and green beans (½ c)					Butter, salad dressing, carbonated beverages

Although we have referred to protein as if it were just one substance, there are actually many different kinds of protein. Proteins are composed of building blocks called **amino acids**; the almost unlimited number of possible combinations and arrangements of amino acids results in many different proteins.

Nine of the 20 amino acids that occur commonly in nature are essential to humans. They are needed for restoring protein levels in your skeletal muscles, blood, skin, hair, heart, enzymes, and in all the other

Amino acids: The building blocks from which proteins are assembled.

Protein quality: The ability of a given food protein to supply the proportions of amino acids needed for synthesizing human protein.

materials in which protein occurs in the body. The nine *essential amino acids* are also needed to form new tissue in people who are still growing, are building muscle, or are pregnant.

Since the amount of essential amino acids (EAAs) present in food varies from one type of food to another, some foods do a better job of meeting your EAA needs than others. Therefore we say that there are differences in **protein quality** among various foods. Eggs and milk are two foods whose proteins are so well-matched to human EAA needs that they are considered the standard to which other food proteins are compared. Foods that compare favorably are said to contain very *high quality* protein.

Meats, fish, poultry, cheese, and soybeans are almost as good as eggs and milk in their essential amino acid patterns; they contain high quality protein also. However, the proteins in most plants offer a less good match; their proteins are of *lower quality*. Finally, gelatin offers a *poor quality* of protein.

People who include foods of both plant and animal origin in their diets do not need to think about whether they are getting adequate amounts of the EAAs; they are likely to be meeting their needs as long as they are getting enough protein overall.

Vegans: Vegetarians who avoid all foods of animal origin, and therefore consume only plant foods.

However, vegetarians who avoid all animal products and eat only plant foods (**vegans**) need to pay more attention to this matter, especially if they are still growing, are pregnant, or lactating. They can get enough of the EAAs if, at the same meal, they eat combinations of various foods such as rice and beans that compensate for the EAA deficiencies of the individual foods.

Generally speaking, legumes (all types of starchy beans and peas) should be the protein mainstays of the vegan diet; and either grain products, nuts, or seeds should be eaten with the legumes at the same meal. This practice is called **complementing** or **mutual supplementation**. Many traditional ethnic food combinations are complementary, such as beans and tortillas, split pea or lentil soup with rye bread, or a tofu (soybean curd) dish with sesame seeds.

Complementing or mutual supplementation: Eating foods together whose amino acid content is proportional to human needs.

Vitamins: a lot from a little

In the early part of this century, vitamins were regarded as wonder substances. People who had been at death's door from vitamin deficiencies such as scurvy or pellagra were restored to excellent health by taking small amounts of these newly isolated substances. Such medical dramas impressed on people the importance of vitamins to health.

Judging from the huge business that vitamin supplement sales represent today, it seems that those early lessons were well learned. Yet, as we mentioned early in the chapter, most people really don't need such supplements. To support that statement, we will provide information about what a vitamin is and does, and which foods contain them.

A vitamin is a noncaloric compound needed in very small amounts for performing regulatory functions that promote growth, permit reproduction, and maintain health and life. Thirteen different vitamins have been identified. They fall into two categories, fat-soluble and water-soluble:

- *Fat-soluble*: vitamins A, D, E, and K
- *Water-soluble*: thiamin, riboflavin, niacin, vitamin B-6, folacin, vitamin B-12, pantothenic acid, biotin, and vitamin C

There are a few other substances that vitamin supplement promoters have marketed as vitamins, but really are not—such as inositol, rutin, para-aminobenzoic acid (PABA), bioflavinoids, lipoic acid, ubiquinone, choline, pangamic acid, and "vitamin B-17" (laetrile). Not only are these substances not vitamins, but the last two on the list can be hazardous.

Vitamins are needed only in milligram (mg) amounts (1 mg equals one-thousandth of a gram); or in microgram (μg) amounts 1 μg equals one-millionth of a gram). A little goes a very long way: with folacin for example, since the recommended intake for adults is 400 μg per day, one gram of folacin would meet the needs of 2500 people for one day.

Table 8.3 summarizes a lot of information about the vitamins: their various names and forms, RDAs, sources, functions, and typical signs of deficiency and excess.

Each vitamin performs its own specific roles in every cell's biochemical activities. Therefore, a vitamin deficiency has widespread effects on the body, even though the most obvious negative signs of deficiency may be more apparent in one part of the body than another. For example, even though a severe deficiency of thiamin is likely to manifest itself most obviously in nervous and muscular disorders, it affects cells throughout the body.

If a person has some signs or symptoms of a vitamin deficiency, he or she should regard them as signals to ask a health care provider for a thorough evaluation. Don't make a judgment yourself: having suspicious symptoms is not proof of having a deficiency, since many other conditions can produce similar effects. Blood and/or urine tests are the most definitive ways to diagnose nutritional deficiencies.

As we have already stated, excessive intakes of vitamins—especially if extreme and/or prolonged—also can have negative effects. For example, the fat-soluble vitamins A and D, taken in excessive amounts, are well known for their toxicity. Other vitamins in high doses are also known to be harmful. There are case reports of people who have developed neuromuscular problems from taking huge doses of vitamin B-6; how ironic it is that the reason they were having trouble with muscular coordination was because they were overdosing themselves with something they thought would benefit them.

Table 8.3   Some facts about vitamins

Vitamin	Alternate names or forms	RDA for healthy adults[a]	Major dietary sources	Major functions	Signs of severe, prolonged deficiency	Signs of extreme excess
Fat-soluble						
A	Retinol Retinal Retinaldehyde Retinoic acid Vitamin A palmitate Carotene	Females: 800 RE, 4000 IU Males: 1000 RE, 5000 IU	Fat-containing and fortified dairy products; liver; carotene in orange and deep green produce	Component of rhodopsin (a substance needed for night vision); still under study	Hardening of the cornea of the eye (may lead to blindness); night blindness; dry, scaling skin; poor immune response	Damage to liver, kidney, bone; headache, irritability, vomiting, hair loss, blurred vision. From carotene: yellowed skin
D	Cholecalciferol Ergocalciferol "The sunshine vitamin"	5 μg (200 IU)	Fortified and full-fat dairy products, egg yolk	Promotes absorption and use of calcium and phosphorus	Rickets (bone deformities) in children; osteomalacia (bone softening) in adults	GI upset; cerebral, vascular, kidney damage; lethargy
E	Tocopherol Tocotrienol	Females: 8 alpha-tocopherol equivalents Males: 10 alpha-tocopherol equivalents	Vegetable oils and their products; nuts, seeds; present at low levels in other foods	Protects cell membrane from damage	Possible anemia	In anemic children, blood abnormalities may develop
K	Phylloquinone Menadione	70–140 μg[b]	Green vegetables; tea; meats	Aids in formation of certain proteins, especially those for blood clotting	Severe bleeding on injury: internal hemorrhage	Liver damage and anemia from high doses of the synthetic form menadione

Continued

Table 8.3 Continued

Vitamin	Alternate names or forms	RDA for healthy adults[a]	Major dietary sources	Major functions	Signs of severe, prolonged deficiency	Signs of extreme excess
Water-soluble						
Thiamin	Vitamin B-1	Females: 1.1 mg Males: 1.5 mg	Pork, legumes, peanuts, enriched or whole grain products	Component of enzyme used in energy metabolism	Beriberi (nerve changes, sometimes edema, heart failure)	?
Riboflavin	Vitamin B-2	Females: 1.3 mg Males: 1.7 mg	Dairy products, meats, eggs, enriched grain products, green leafy vegetables	Component of enzyme used in energy metabolism	Skin lesions	?
Niacin	Nicotinamide Nicotinic acid	Females: 14 niacin equivalents Males: 19 niacin equivalents	Nuts, meats; most proteins	Component of coenzyme used in energy metabolism	Pellagra (diarrhea, dermatitis, dementia, death)	Flushing of face, neck, hands; liver damage
B-6	Pyridoxine Pyridoxamine Pyridoxal Pyridoxol	Females: 2.0 mg Males: 2.2 mg	High protein foods in general, bananas, some vegetables	Component of coenzyme used in amino acid metabolism	Nervous and muscular disorders	Unstable gait, numb feet, poor hand coordination, abnormal brain function
Folacin	Folic acid Folate Pteroylglutamic acid	400 μg	Green vegetables, orange juice, nuts, legumes, grain products	Component of coenzyme used in DNA and RNA metabolism	Anemia; GI disturbances	Masks vitamin B-12 deficiency
B-12	Cobalamin Cyanocobalamin	3 μg	Animal products	Component of coenzyme used in DNA and RNA metabolism	Anemia; nervous system damage	?

Continued

Table 8.3 Continued

Vitamin	Alternate names or forms	RDA for healthy adults[a]	Major dietary sources	Major functions	Signs of severe, prolonged deficiency	Signs of extreme excess
Water-soluble (Continued)						
Pantothenic acid	Pantothenate	4–7 mg[b]	Widely distributed in foods	Component of coenzyme used in energy metabolism	Fatigue, sleep disturbances, nausea, poor coordination	?
Biotin		100–200 µg[b]	Widely distributed in foods	Component of coenzyme used in energy metabolism	Fatigue, depression, muscular pain, dermatitis	?
C	Ascorbic acid Ascorbate	60 mg	Fruits and vegetables, especially broccoli, cabbage, cantaloupe, cauliflower, citrus fruits, green pepper, strawberries	Maintains connective tissue; protects against oxidation; aids in detoxification; still under study	Scurvy (skin spots, bleeding gums, weakness); delayed wound healing; impaired immune response	GI upsets, confounds certain lab tests, poorer immune response

[a]Recommended Dietary Allowances (RDAs) are amounts of nutrients recommended for average daily intake by normally healthy people in the United States. These were published in 1980.
[b]Estimated Safe and Adequate Daily Dietary Intakes (1980).

Now let's focus on the original (and still the best) source of vitamins—food. Vitamins are widely distributed in foods by nature. Some vitamins (e.g., pantothenic acid and biotin) occur in almost all foods, so people are virtually assured of getting enough of them in their diets. Other vitamins are present in significant amounts only in particular types of foods (e.g., vitamin C in fruits and vegetables, and vitamin B-12 in foods of animal origin), so people need to be more deliberate about eating the foods that contain them.

Scan the column of major dietary sources in Table 8.3. You will see that if you consume fruits and vegetables, meat and legumes, grain products, and dairy products, you are likely to take in all of the vitamins in some amount. This should reassure you if you are concerned about vitamin deficiency.

On the other hand, of all the categories of nutrients, vitamins are the most fragile. Some vitamins break down at a particular acidity or alkalinity, others in light, or from heat. All gradually lose their potency with time. Therefore food that is old, or has been carelessly stored, or has been highly processed has lost some of its original vitamin value.

Commercial processors are aware of the conditions that can cause vitamin loss. They know that vitamin levels are lowered when grains are refined (stripped of their outer, nutrient-rich bran layers) or when foods are frozen, canned, dried, or cooked. Therefore, they have modified many of their processes to minimize nutrient losses.

To compensate for losses of low levels in some foods, vitamins (and sometimes other nutrients) are added in small amounts to foods, a process called **fortification**. A common type of fortification is **enrichment**, in which the vitamins thiamin, riboflavin, niacin, and the mineral iron are added to refined grain products. You can tell which breads, cereals, pastas, white flour, and other items have been enriched because they must be so labeled.

Even though vitamins are vulnerable to destruction, it is relatively easy to consume sufficient amounts of vitamins from foods by following some simple dietary guidelines. We will offer such recommendations in the chapter on nutrition programs, Chapter 10, along with suggestions about how to handle and prepare food at home in ways that will retain the most nutrients.

Fortification: Any addition of nutrients to foods in the course of processing.

Enrichment: The addition of nutrients already present in a food, raising them to standard levels specified by the U.S. Food and Drug Administration.

Minerals: the elemental essentials

Minerals, like vitamins, are noncaloric substances needed in small amounts. They are different from vitamins in that minerals are single elements only, whereas vitamins are compounds of carbon, hydrogen, oxygen, and sometimes other elements as well. There are 21 minerals thought to be needed by humans; however, since this is still a very active area of research, it is possible that other essential minerals may be identified in the future.

Minerals are usually classified in two groups, depending on the relative amounts present in the body. Those present in larger amounts—and therefore needed in larger amounts in the diet—are called *major minerals*. Those present in smaller amounts are called *trace minerals*. The minerals included in each category are as follows:

- *Major minerals*: calcium, phosphorus, sulfur, potassium, chloride, sodium, magnesium
- *Trace minerals*: iron, iodine, fluoride, zinc, selenium, copper, cobalt, chromium, manganese, molybdenum, arsenic, nickel, silicon, vanadium

The mineral table (Table 8.4) identifies many of the essential minerals' recommended intakes, dietary sources, major functions, signs of deficiency, and signs of excess. Looking at their functions, you can see that minerals give hardness to bones and teeth. In addition, minerals serve many regulatory functions, such as binding oxygen to the blood protein hemoglobin, and influencing body water distribution.

Table 8.4 Some facts about minerals

Mineral	RDA for healthy adults[a]	Major dietary sources	Major functions	Signs of severe, prolonged deficiency	Signs of extreme excess
Major minerals					
Calcium	800 mg	Milk, cheese, dark green vegetables, legumes	Bone and tooth formation; blood clotting; nerve transmission	Stunted growth; maybe bone loss	Depressed absorption of some other minerals
Phosphorus	800 mg	Milk, cheese, meat, poultry, whole grains	Bone and tooth formation; acid-base balance; component of enzymes	Weakness; demineralization of bone	Depressed absorption of some minerals
Magnesium	Females: 300 mg Males: 350 mg	Whole grains, green leafy vegetables	Component of enzymes	Neurological disturbances	Neurological disturbances
Sulfur	(Provided by sulfur amino acids)	Sulfur amino acids in dietary proteins	Component of cartilage, tendon, and proteins; acid-base balance	Stunted growth, weakness, impaired immune function	Excess sulfur amino acid intake leads to poor growth; liver damage
Sodium	1100–3300 mg[b]	Salt, soy sauce, cured meats, pickles, canned soups, processed cheese	Body water balance; nerve function	Muscle cramps; reduced appetite	High blood pressure in genetically predisposed individuals
Potassium	1875–5625 mg[b]	Meats, milk, many fruits and vegetables, whole grains	Body water balance; nerve function	Muscular weakness; paralysis	Muscular weakness; cardiac arrest
Chloride	1700–5100 mg[b]	Salt, many processed foods (as for sodium)	Plays a role in acid-base balance; formation of gastric juice	Muscle cramps; reduced appetite; poor growth	Vomiting

Continued

Table 8.4 Continued

Mineral	RDA for healthy adults[a]	Major dietary sources	Major functions	Signs of severe, prolonged deficiency	Signs of extreme excess
Trace minerals					
Iron	Females: 18 mg Males: 10 mg	Meats, eggs, legumes, whole grains, green leafy vegetables	Component of hemoglobin (a blood protein), myoglobin (a muscle protein), and enzymes	Iron deficiency anemia, weakness, impaired immune function	Acute: shock, death Chronic: liver damage, cardiac failure
Iodine	0.15 mg	Marine fish and shellfish; dairy products; iodized salt; some breads	Component of thyroid hormones	Goiter (enlarged thyroid)	Iodide goiter
Fluoride	1.5–4.0 mg[b]	Drinking water, tea, seafood	Maintenance of tooth (and maybe bone) structure	Higher frequency of tooth decay	Mottling of teeth; skeletal deformation
Zinc	15 mg	Meats, seafood, whole grains	Component of enzymes	Growth failure; reproductive failure; impaired immune function	Acute: nausea; vomiting; diarrhea. Chronic: adversely affects copper metabolism and immune function
Selenium	0.05–0.2 mg[b]	Seafood, meat, whole grains	Component of enzyme; functions in close association with vitamin E	Muscle pain; maybe heart muscle deterioration	Hair and nail loss
Copper	2–3 mg[b]	Seafood, nuts, legumes, organ meats	Component of enzymes	Anemia; bone and cardiovascular changes	Liver and neurological damage
Cobalt	(Required as vitamin B-12)	Vitamin B-12 (animal products)	Component of vitamin B-12	Not reported except as vitamin B-12 deficiency	With alcohol: heart failure

Continued

Table 8.4 Continued

Mineral	RDA for healthy adults[a]	Major dietary sources	Major functions	Signs of severe, prolonged deficiency	Signs of extreme excess
Trace minerals (Continued)					
Chromium	0.05–0.2 mg[b]	Brewers' yeast, liver, seafood, meat, some vegetables	Involved in glucose and energy metabolism	Impaired glucose metabolism	Lung, skin, and kidney damage (occupational exposures)
Manganese	2.5–5.0 mg[b]	Nuts, whole grains, vegetables and fruits	Component of enzymes	Abnormal bone and cartilage	Neuro-muscular effects
Molybdenum	0.15–0.5 mg[b]	Legumes, cereals, some vegetables	Component of enzymes	Disorder in nitrogen excretion	Inhibition of enzymes; adversely affects cobalt metabolism

[a]Recommended Dietary Allowances (RDAs) are amounts of nutrients recommended for average daily intake by normally healthy people in the United States. These were published in 1980.
[b]Estimated Safe and Adequate Daily Dietary Intakes (1980).

Minerals are widely distributed in the food supply; however, there is no one food that contains all the essential minerals, nor is there a mineral that is found in large amounts in all foods; this underlines the importance of a varied diet. However, some minerals are more concentrated in certain types of foods, such as calcium in dairy products, and iron in meats.

Furthermore, there can be considerable variation in the mineral contents of different samples of a given plant food, depending on the mineral content of the soil, water, and/or fertilizer used for growing the plant. This is true especially for iodine, fluoride, and selenium.

Because of the scarcity of iodine in soils in certain parts of the country, the iodine content of plants grown there is very low. In the past, when people consumed foods mainly grown locally, iodine deficiency, or goiter, was a serious public health problem; in regions of low-soil-iodine content, this led to the practice of adding iodine to salt to assure adequate intake of this mineral. Now, however, iodine is generously available from certain additives, so iodine deficiency is unlikely in the United States.

There are other noteworthy instances of how processing changes the level of minerals in foods. Just as the refinement of grains brings about a number of vitamin losses, it also substantially decreases mineral content. One of the minerals most affected is iron, which is of particular concern because iron is also the mineral most likely to be in short supply in American diets, especially for women. Fortunately, iron is restored if the grain is enriched at a later processing stage, but the many other minerals that were lost are not replaced.

Sodium and chloride are minerals that are commonly added to food by the widespread practice of salting. One example of how salting affects the sodium content of food is shown by comparing fresh vegetables with canned soups made from them. Whereas fresh vegetables generally have less than 10 mg of sodium per serving, a cup of commercially canned vegetable soup may contain 1000 mg. This is of concern from a health standpoint; the high sodium content of the typical American diet may promote high blood pressure in susceptible individuals. (This will be discussed when we deal with cardiovascular disease in a later chapter.)

There is yet another concern about mineral nutrition. The question is: How much of the mineral present in a food will ultimately be useful to the body? The degree to which the body is able to use a substance in the form actually present is called its **bioavailability**. Bioavailability is more of a concern for minerals than for any other class of nutrients.

Bioavailability: Degree to which the body is able to use a substance in the form actually present.

Iron serves as a good example. Scientists have learned that iron is used by the body with different efficiency depending on the food. Overall, about 10 percent of the iron present in foods is absorbed, but the absorption rate averages around 25 percent from meats and may be as low as 2 percent from some plant foods. This is because there are factors in meat that enhance the absorption of iron from it, and there are factors in plants that interfere with absorption.

Fortunately, we now know the following ways to increase the absorption rate of iron from plant sources by as much as twofold:

- Consume a good source of vitamin C, such as orange juice, at the same meal as the plant source of iron.
- Include some meat in the same meal as the plant source of iron.

Although iron represents the most extreme example of low bioavailability, there are also dietary factors known to influence the body's utilization of calcium, phosphorus, magnesium, and zinc. This is of particular concern for vegans, because their diets normally contain greater amounts of the factors which interfere with mineral absorption.

People who eat both plant and animal products usually can absorb the amount of minerals they need from their diets alone; supplements are not generally necessary. In fact, we usually discourage mineral supplementation because the human body is quite sensitive to mineral overdoses. Table 8.4 points out some consequences of toxic doses. As with vitamins, we encourage people to get the minerals they need from food by following the food guide in Chapter 10.

Nonetheless, there are some instances in which supplements may be in order, such as iron for women, who are at greater risk for iron-deficiency anemia due to menstrual losses of blood, or who often need extra iron during pregnancy. Calcium supplements are receiving much commercial promotion as a protection against osteoporosis, but such supplements are probably of limited benefit. This is discussed more thoroughly in Chapter 13.

Now that you have a firm grounding in the basics of nutrition, you are ready to assess your own diet as described in the next chapter.

How to Evaluate Your Diet 9

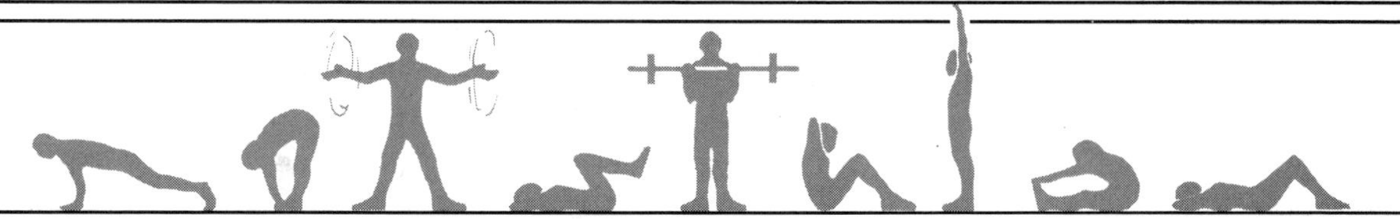

Outline

Mike thinks of himself as a meat-and-potatoes man: he likes fairly plain foods, drinks whole milk, eats a lot of bread and other baked goods, and only occasionally includes salads or cooked vegetables with his meals. He commonly snacks on potato or corn chips, and sometimes on apples or bananas.

Beth has a different eating style. Always conscious of her weight, she tries to avoid starchy foods, except for the bowl of cereal or piece of toast she has in the morning. For the rest of the day, she emphasizes meats, fruits, vegetables, and salads with low-calorie dressing. She drinks lots of diet soda between meals. When she adheres to this diet, she often feels hungry and craves sweet and starchy foods; every two or three days she satisfies her cravings by eating ice cream, chocolate chip cookies, or caramel corn . . . or all three.

Aaron has different likes and dislikes. He has chosen a lacto-ovo-vegetarian eating style: he eats dairy products, eggs, and plant products (fruits, vegetables, grains, nuts, seeds). Mainstays of his diet are macaroni and cheese, peanut butter sandwiches, and meatless Oriental entrees; he avoids all meats, fish, and poultry.

Julie likes most kinds of foods, and likes to try new things. She enjoys

145

Self-check 9.1   Documenting your food and nutrient intakes for one day

1. List the foods and amounts you consumed during one day in the first two columns of the form below.
2. Get data for other columns from Table 9.1, adjusting the energy and nutrient values for the size of serving that you actually consumed.
3. If you are using data from food product labels, follow instructions for converting percent of the U.S. RDA into absolute values as described in the text.
4. Determine the total value for each column.

Items consumed	Amount	Energy (kcal)	Protein (grams)	Fat (grams)	Carbohydrate (grams)	Iron (mg)	Calcium (mg)	Sodium (mg)	Vitamin A (IU)	Thiamin (vitamin B-1) (mg)	Riboflavin (vitamin B-2) (mg)	Niacin (mg)	Vitamin C (ascorbic acid) (mg)
Total													

Tr = trace
— = data are unreliable

all of the kinds of foods eaten by Mike, Beth, and Aaron, but wouldn't want to be limited to any one of those eating styles.

Whose diet is the healthiest?

This chapter provides methods you can use to evaluate these different kinds of eating patterns—and, of course, to evaluate your own diet as well. From the information in this chapter, you will be able to assess how close your diet comes to the recommended intakes for energy, protein, vitamins and minerals, and what proportion of kcalories you get from each energy source.

Documenting the Way You Eat

Before you can analyze your diet, you need to have a listing of what (and how much) you eat on a typical day.

One way to collect this information is to keep a food record. Simply write down all the foods, beverages, and supplements you consume in the course of a day, as well as the amount of each item. The first two columns of Self-check 9.1 provide a convenient format, and Figure 9.1 shows an example of a filled-out form. Don't forget the details— the mayonnaise on the sandwich, the butter used to fry the egg, the dressing on the salad. Estimating amounts accurately takes some practice; measure out a few servings of various foods and look at those amounts on the dish you'd eat them from; this can help you develop an eye for quantities.

Keep your intake as typical as possible on a day you are recording. Sometimes when people keep a food record, they are tempted to change their eating to reflect what they think they *ought* to eat instead of what they usually *do* eat. Try to resist this temptation so that you will get meaningful information.

You will get a more accurate picture of your overall intake if you analyze several consecutive days instead of just one. Record at least two days during the week as well as one during the weekend, since your intake on those days may be quite different.

Calculating Your Nutrient Intake

Next, you need to know what levels of nutrients were in the substances you consumed. Such information is available for thousands of items on tables of food composition and in computerized nutrient data banks.

The U.S. Department of Agriculture (USDA) has been the leader in the United States in assembling food composition information. Table 9.1 provides USDA data for approximately 200 items that are commonly consumed in this country. Use this table to look up the items on your record, and fill in the values for energy and the nutrients, adjusting them if you ate an amount which differs from the amount given in the table. For example, if you drank 1/2 cup of milk but the

Text continued on page 160.

Figure 9.1   An example of using Self-check 9.1 to document your food and nutrient intakes for one day. This example involves Lori, an 18-year-old, full-grown student who gets moderate exercise.

1. List the foods and amounts you consumed during one day in the first two columns of the form below.
2. Get data for other columns from Table 9.1, adjusting the energy and nutrient values for the size of serving that you actually consumed.
3. If you are using data from food product labels, follow instructions for converting percent of the U.S. RDA into absolute values as described in the text.
4. Determine the total value for each column.

Items consumed	Amount	Energy (kcal)	Protein (grams)	Fat (grams)	Carbohydrate (grams)	Iron (mg)	Calcium (mg)	Sodium (mg)	Vitamin A (IU)	Thiamin (vitamin B-1) (mg)	Riboflavin (vitamin B-2) (mg)	Niacin (mg)	Vitamin C (ascorbic acid) (mg)
Cornflakes, fortified	1 cup	97	2.0	0.1	21.3	0.6	—	251	1180	.29	.35	2.9	9
Milk, 2%	½ cup	61	4.1	2.4	5.9	0.1	149	61	250	.05	.20	.1	1
Sugar	1 T.	46	0	0	12.0	Tr	0	Tr	0	0	0	0	0
Cola	12 oz. can	144	0	0	36.9	0	0	—	0	0	0	0	0
Soup, cream of mushroom	½ can	166	2.9	11.9	12.5	0.5	51	1185	90	.02	.15	0.9	Tr
Sandwich: Bread, white enr.	2 slices	148	4.8	2.0	27.2	1.4	52	268	Tr	.14	.10	1.2	Tr
Luncheon meat (salami values)	2 oz.	256	13.4	21.6	.6	2.0	8	—	—	.20	.14	3.0	—
Mayonnaise	1 T.	101	0.2	11.2	.3	0.1	3	84	40	Tr	.01	Tr	—
Coffee	10 oz.	negligible											→
Cookies, vanilla wafers	10	139	1.6	4.8	22.3	0.1	12	76	40	.01	.02	.1	0
Milk, 2%	1 cup	121	8.1	4.7	11.7	0.1	297	122	500	.10	.40	.2	2
Spaghetti, cnd., w/ meatballs, sce.	1 cup	258	12.3	10.3	28.5	3.3	53	1220	1000	.15	.18	2.3	5
Bread, French, enr.	1 slice	73	2.3	.8	13.9	0.6	11	145	Tr	.07	.06	.6	Tr
Butter	½ T.	51	0.1	5.8	.1	0	2	70	235	—	—	—	0
Lettuce	1 cup	7	0.5	.1	1.6	0.3	11	5	180	.03	.03	.2	3
Salad dressing, Italian	2 T.	166	Tr	18.0	2.0	Tr	4	628	Tr	Tr	Tr	Tr	—
Popcorn	4 cups	92	3.2	1.2	18.4	0.8	4	Tr	—	.04	.40	0	0
w/ butter	2 T.	204	0.2	23.0	.2	0	6	280	940	—	—	—	0
Soft drink, orange (cola values)	12 oz.	144	0	0	36.9	0	0	—	0	0	0	0	0
Total		2274	55.7	117.9	252.3	9.9	663	4395	4455	1.10	2.04	11.5	20

Tr = trace
— = data are unreliable

Table 9.1 Composition of various foods

Food	Serving size	Food energy (kcal)	Protein (g)	Fat (g)	Carbo-hydrate (g)	Iron (mg)[a]	Cal-cium (mg)	So-dium (mg)	Vit. A (IU)[b]	Thia-min (mg)	Riboflavin (mg)	Niacin (mg)	Vit. C (mg)
Almonds	10 nuts	60	1.9	5.4	2.0	0.5	23	6	0	.02	.09	.4	Trace
Apples (3 per lb.)	1 medium	80	0.3	.8	20.0	0.4	10	1	120	.04	.03	.1	6
Apple juice	6 oz	87	0.2	Trace	22.1	1.1	11	2	—[c]	.02	.04	.2	2
Applesauce, un-sweetened	1 cup	100	0.5	.5	26.4	1.2	10	5	100	.05	.02	.1	2
Apricots, canned	1 cup	93	1.7	.2	23.6	0.7	30	2	4500	.05	.05	1.0	10
Asparagus, canned	1 cup	44	4.6	.7	7.1	4.1	44	576	1240	.15	.22	2.0	37
Avocado	1/2 fruit	188	2.4	18.5	7.1	0.7	11	5	330	.12	.23	1.8	16
Bacon, 20 sl/lb, raw	2 slices	86	3.8	7.8	.5	0.5	2	153	0	.08	.05	.8	—
Bananas, medium	1 banana	101	1.3	.2	26.4	0.8	10	1	230	.06	.07	.8	12
Beans & frank-furters	1 cup	367	19.4	18.1	32.1	4.8	94	1374	330	.18	.15	3.3	Trace
Beef, boneless chuck, lean (braised/ stewed)	1 cup	300	42.0	13.3	0	5.3	18	74	20	.08	.32	6.4	—
Beef & vegetable stew, canned	1 cup	194	14.2	7.6	17.4	2.2	29	1007	2380	.07	.12	2.5	7
Beer, 4.5% alco-hol	12-oz can	151	1.1	0	13.7	Trace	18	25	—	.01	.11	2.2	—
Beets, cooked	1 cup, diced or sliced	54	1.9	.2	12.2	0.9	24	73	30	.05	.07	.5	10
Beet greens, cooked	1 cup	26	2.5	.3	4.8	2.8	144	110	7400	.10	.22	.4	22
Biscuit, enriched	1 biscuit, 2-in di-ameter	103	2.1	4.8	12.8	0.4	34	175	Trace	.06	.06	.5	Trace
Blueberries, raw	1 cup	90	1.0	.7	22.2	1.5	22	1	150	.04	.09	.7	20
Bologna	1 slice, 1 oz	86	3.4	7.8	.3	0.5	2	369	—	.05	.06	.7	—

Table 9.1 (Continued)

Food	Serving size	Food energy (kcal)	Protein (g)	Fat (g)	Carbo-hydrate (g)	Iron (mg)[a]	Cal-cium (mg)	So-dium (mg)	Vit. A (IU)[b]	Thia-min (mg)	Riboflavin (mg)	Niacin (mg)	Vit. C (mg)
Bread: Cracked wheat	1 slice, 1 oz	66	2.2	.6	13.0	0.3	22	132	Trace	.03	.02	.3	Trace
French, en-riched	1 slice, 1 oz	73	2.3	.8	13.9	0.6	11	145	Trace	.07	.06	.6	Trace
Raisin, enriched	1 slice, 1 oz	66	1.7	.7	13.4	0.3	18	91	Trace	.01	.02	.2	Trace
Rye	1 slice, 1 oz	61	2.3	.3	13.0	0.4	19	139	0	.05	.02	.4	0
White, enriched	1 slice, 1 oz	74	2.4	1.0	13.6	0.7	26	134	Trace	.07	.05	.6	Trace
Whole wheat	1 slice, 1 oz	61	2.6	.8	11.9	0.8	25	132	Trace	.06	.03	.7	Trace
Broccoli, frozen, chopped	10 oz	82	9.1	.9	14.8	2.0	165	48	7380	.20	.37	1.7	200
Brownie, commer-cial	1, 1 oz	117	1.4	5.8	17.2	0.5	11	57	57	.06	.02	.08	Trace
Butter	1 tbsp	102	0.1	11.5	.1	0	3	140	470	—	—	—	0
Buttermilk, from skim	1 cup	88	8.8	.2	12.5	0.1	296	319	10	.10	.44	.2	2
Cabbage, raw, shredded	1 cup	17	0.9	.1	3.8	0.3	34	14	90	.04	.04	.2	33
Cake: Angel food	1 slice, 1 oz	81	2.1	.1	18.1	0.1	3	85	0	Trace	.04	.1	0
Chocolate cup-cake, uniced	1, 1 oz	103	1.3	4.3	20.4	0.2	21	92	45	.01	.03	.1	Trace
Candy: Milk chocolate	1 oz	147	2.2	9.2	16.1	0.3	65	27	80	.02	.10	.1	Trace
Jellybeans	1 oz (10)	104	Trace	.1	26.4	0.3	3	3	0	0	Trace	Trace	0
Cantaloupe	1 c., 20 balls	48	1.1	.2	12.0	0.6	22	19	5440	.06	.05	1.0	53
Carrots, raw	1, 3 oz	30	0.8	.1	7.0	0.5	27	34	7930	.04	.04	.4	6
Cashew nuts, roasted in oil	1 oz	159	4.9	13.0	8.3	1.1	11	4	30	.12	.07	.5	—
Catsup	1 tbsp	16	0.3	.1	3.8	0.1	3	156	210	.01	.01	.2	, 2
Cauliflower, raw, chopped	1 cup	31	3.1	.2	6.0	1.3	29	15	70	.13	.12	.8	90
Celery, raw, chopped	1 cup	20	1.1	.1	4.7	0.4	47	151	320	.04	.04	.4	11

Food	Serving size	Food energy (kcal)	Protein (g)	Fat (g)	Carbo-hydrate (g)	Iron (mg)[a]	Cal-cium (mg)	So-dium (mg)	Vit. A (IU)[b]	Thia-min (mg)	Riboflavin (mg)	Niacin (mg)	Vit. C (mg)
Cheese: American	1 slice, 1 oz	100	6.3	8.1	.5	0.2	188	307	330	.01	.11	Trace	0
Cheddar	1 oz	113	7.1	9.1	.6	0.3	213	198	370	.01	.13	Trace	0
Cottage, small curd	1 cup	223	28.6	8.8	6.1	0.6	197	481	360	.06	.53	.2	0
Parmesan, shredded	1 tbsp	21	1.9	1.4	.2	Trace	61	39	60	Trace	.04	Trace	0
Swiss	1 oz	105	7.8	7.9	.5	0.3	262	201	320	Trace	.11	Trace	0
Cheese food/ spread	1 tbsp	40	2.2	3.0	1.1	0.1	79	228	120	Trace	.08	Trace	0
Cherries, sweet, raw	10 cher-ries	47	0.9	.2	11.7	0.3	15	1	70	.03	.04	.4	7
Chicken, light meat	2 oz	94	17.9	1.9	0	0.7	6	36	34	.02	.06	6.6	—
Dark meat	2 oz	100	15.9	3.6	0	1.0	7	49	84	.04	.13	3.2	—
Chili with beans, canned	1 cup	339	19.1	15.6	31.1	4.3	82	1354	150	.08	.18	3.3	—
Chow mein, canned, chicken, w/o noodles	1 cup	95	6.5	.3	17.8	1.3	45	725	150	.05	.10	1.0	13
Clams, canned, minced	1 cup	157	25.3	4.0	3.0	—	—	—	—	—	—	—	—
Collards, frozen, chopped	10 oz con-tainer	91	8.8	1.1	16.5	3.1	542	51	19310	.20	.45	2.0	193
Cookies: Choc. chip	1 oz	138	1.5	8.1	19.2	.8	9	63	12	.06	.06	0.3	0
Fig bar	2 oz, 4 cookies	200	2.2	3.1	42.2	0.6	44	141	60	.02	.04	.2	Trace
Vanilla wafers	1 oz, 10 cookies	139	1.6	4.8	22.3	0.1	12	76	40	.01	.02	.1	0
Corn, canned, sol-ids	1 cup	139	4.3	1.3	32.7	0.8	8	389	580	.05	.08	1.5	7
Creamed	1 cup	210	5.4	1.5	51.2	1.5	8	604	840	.08	.13	2.6	13
On-the-cob	1 5-in ear	70	2.5	.8	16.2	0.5	2	Trace	310	.09	.08	1.1	7

Table 9.1   (Continued)

Food	Serving size	Food energy (kcal)	Protein (g)	Fat (g)	Carbo-hydrate (g)	Iron (mg)[a]	Cal-cium (mg)	So-dium (mg)	Vit. A (IU)[b]	Thia-min (mg)	Riboflavin (mg)	Niacin (mg)	Vit. C (mg)
Corn bread, from mix	2 oz	178	3.8	5.8	27.5	0.8	133	263	130	.10	.10	.8	Trace
Corn flakes, forti-fied	1 cup	97	2.0	.1	21.3	0.6	—	251	1180	.29	.35	2.9	9
Corn grits, cooked, en-riched	1 cup	125	2.9	.2	27.0	0.2	2	502	150	.05	.02	.5	0
Corned beef, canned	2 oz	123	14.3	6.8	0	2.4	11	—	—	.01	.14	1.9	0
Corned beef hash, canned	1 cup	398	19.4	24.9	23.5	4.4	29	1188	—	.02	.20	4.6	—
Corn flakes, forti-fied	1 cup	97	2.0	.1	21.3	0.6	—	251	1180	.29	.35	2.9	9
Crackers, graham	2, 2½ in sq.	55	1.1	1.3	10.4	0.2	6	95	0	.01	.03	.2	0
Saltine	10 crack-ers	123	2.6	3.4	20.3	0.3	6	312	0	Trace	.01	.3	0
Cranberry juice cocktail	1 cup	164	0.3	.3	41.7	0.8	13	3	Trace	.03	.03	.1	40
Cream, half 'n half	1 tbsp	20	0.5	1.8	.7	Trace	16	7	70	Trace	.02	Trace	Trace
Sour half 'n half	1 tbsp	20	Trace	1.8	.6	Trace	14	6	68	Trace	.02	Trace	Trace
Whipped top-ping	1 tbsp	11	Trace	.9	.6	Trace	3	2	19	0	0	0	0
Cucumbers, raw, sliced	1 cup	16	0.9	.1	3.6	1.2	26	6	260	.03	.04	.2	12
Dandelion greens, cooked	1 cup	35	2.1	.6	6.7	1.9	147	46	12290	.14	.17	—	19
Dates	10 dates	219	1.8	.4	58.3	2.4	47	1	40	.07	.08	1.8	0
Doughnut, cake, plain	1, 2 oz	227	2.7	10.8	29.8	0.8	23	291	50	.09	.09	.7	Trace
Egg, raw	1 large	82	6.5	5.8	.5	1.2	27	61	590	.05	.15	Trace	0
Fish stick	1 stick, 1 oz	50	4.7	2.5	1.8	0.1	3	—	0	.01	.02	.5	—

Food	Serving size	Food energy (kcal)	Protein (g)	Fat (g)	Carbohydrate (g)	Iron (mg)[a]	Calcium (mg)	Sodium (mg)	Vit. A (IU)[b]	Thiamin (mg)	Riboflavin (mg)	Niacin (mg)	Vit. C (mg)
Frankfurter/hot dog	1, 2 oz	176	7.1	15.7	1.0	1.1	4	627	—	.09	.11	1.5	—
Fruit cocktail, canned in heavy syrup	1 cup	194	1.0	.3	50.2	1.0	23	13	360	.05	.03	1.0	5
Gelatin dessert	1 cup	142	3.6	0	33.8	—	—	122	—	—	—	—	—
Gingerbread	1 in cube	17	0.2	.4	3.1	0.1	5	19	Trace	Trace	.01	Trace	Trace
Grapefruit pieces	1 cup	72	0.9	.2	18.6	0.7	28	2	140	.07	.04	.4	67
Grapefruit juice, unsweetened	6 oz	76	0.9	.2	18.2	0.2	19	2	20	.08	.03	.4	72
Grapes, Thompson, seedless	1 cup	107	1.0	.5	27.7	0.6	19	5	160	.08	.05	.5	6
Grape juice	6 oz	125	0.4	Trace	31.5	0.6	21	4	—	.08	.04	.4	Trace
Green beans, canned	1 cup	43	2.4	.2	10.0	2.9	81	564	690	.07	.10	.7	10
Haddock, oven-fried	1 fillet, 4 oz	182	21.6	7.0	6.4	1.3	44	195	—	.04	.08	3.5	2
Halibut, broiled with butter	1 fillet, 4½ oz	214	31.5	8.8	0	1.0	20	168	850	.06	.09	10.4	—
Ham, baked	3 oz	318	19.6	26.0	0	2.6	9	48	0	.43	.20	3.9	—
Hamburger patty med. fat, cooked	3 oz	224	21.8	14.5	0	3.3	6	40	0	.13	.15	4.8	0
Honey	1 tbsp	64	0.1	0	17.3	0.1	1	1	0	Trace	.01	.1	Trace
Ice cream, 10% fat	1 cup	257	6.0	14.1	27.7	0.1	194	84	590	.05	.28	.1	1
Ice milk, 5% fat, hardened	1 cup, 8 oz	199	6.3	6.7	29.3	0.1	204	89	280	.07	.29	.1	1
Ice milk, 5% fat, soft-serve	1 cup, 8 oz	266	8.4	8.9	39.2	0.2	273	119	370	.09	.39	.2	2
Jam	1 tbsp	54	0.1	Trace	14.0	0.2	4	2	Trace	Trace	Trace	Trace	Trace
Jelly	1 tbsp	49	Trace	Trace	12.7	0.3	4	3	Trace	Trace	.01	Trace	1
Kale, cooked	1 cup	43	5.0	.8	6.7	1.8	206	47	9130	.11	.20	1.8	102

Table 9.1 (Continued)

Food	Serving size	Food energy (kcal)	Protein (g)	Fat (g)	Carbo-hydrate (g)	Iron (mg)[a]	Cal-cium (mg)	So-dium (mg)	Vit. A (IU)[b]	Thia-min (mg)	Riboflavin (mg)	Niacin (mg)	Vit. C (mg)
Lamb, broiled chop	2½oz cooked wt (4 per lb)	255	5.6	20.9	0	0.9	6	38	—	.09	.16	3.6	—
Lard	1 tbsp	117	0	13.0	0	0	0	0	0	0	0	0	0
Lasagna, cheese	8 oz	300	12.0	12.0	35.0	2.5	227	670	837	.18	.27	2.2	0
Lemon, 2¼-in diam.	1 lemon	24	1.0	.3	7.1	0.5	23	2	20	.03	.02	.1	46
Lettuce, raw, chopped or shredded	1 cup	7	0.5	.1	1.6	0.3	11	5	180	.03	.03	.2	3
Lima beans, fro-zen, cooked	1 cup	168	10.2	.2	32.5	2.9	34	172	390	.12	.09	1.7	29
Liver, beef, fried	3 oz	195	22.4	9.0	4.5	7.5	9	156	45390	.22	3.56	14.0	23
Liverwurst	1 oz	90	4.2	7.8	.7	1.7	3	—	1850	.05	.41	2.3	—
Lunchmeat, boiled ham	1 oz	66	5.4	4.8	0	0.8	3	—	0	.12	.04	.7	—
Macaroni/cheese, canned	1 cup	228	9.4	9.6	25.7	1.0	199	730	260	.12	.24	1.0	Trace
Macaroni, en-riched, cooked	1 cup	192	6.5	.7	39.1	1.4	14	1	0	.23	.13	1.8	0
Margarine,	1 tbsp	102	0.1	11.5	.1	0	3	140	470	—	—	—	0
Mayonnaise	1 tbsp	101	0.2	11.2	.3	0.1	3	84	40	Trace	.01	Trace	—
Milk, whole, 3.5%	1 cup	159	8.5	8.5	12.0	0.1	288	122	350	.07	.41	.2	2
Low-fat, 2%	1 cup	121	8.1	4.7	11.7	.1	297	122	500	.10	.40	.2	2
Skim	1 cup	88	8.8	.2	12.5	0.1	296	127	10	.09	.44	.2	2
Chocolate, whole	1 cup	213	8.5	8.5	27.5	0.5	278	118	330	.08	.40	.3	3
Evaporated	1 cup	345	17.6	19.9	24.4	0.3	635	297	810	.10	.86	.5	3
Molasses, me-dium	1 tbsp	46	—	—	12.0	1.2	58	7	—	—	.02	.2	—

Food	Serving size	Food energy (kcal)	Protein (g)	Fat (g)	Carbohydrate (g)	Iron (mg)[a]	Calcium (mg)	Sodium (mg)	Vit. A (IU)[b]	Thiamin (mg)	Riboflavin (mg)	Niacin (mg)	Vit. C (mg)
Muffin, from mix	1 muffin (¼ cup batter)	130	2.8	4.2	20.0	0.6	96	192	100	.07	.08	.6	Trace
Mushroom, fresh, slices	1 cup	20	1.9	.2	3.1	0.6	4	11	Trace	.07	.32	2.9	2
Mustard, yellow	1 tsp	4	0.2	.2	.3	0.1	4	63	—	—	—	—	—
Mustard greens, boiled	1 cup	32	3.1	.6	5.6	2.5	193	25	8120	.11	.20	.8	67
Noodles, egg, cooked, enriched	1 cup	200	6.6	2.4	37.3	1.4	16	3	110	.22	.13	1.9	0
Chow mein	1 cup	220	5.9	10.6	26.1	—	—	—	—	—	—	—	—
Oatmeal, cooked	1 cup	133	4.8	2.4	23.3	1.4	22	523	0	.19	.05	.2	0
Ocean perch, breaded, frozen	1 fillet, 3 oz	281	16.6	16.6	14.5	—	—	—	—	—	—	—	—
Oil, corn	1 tbsp	120	0	13.6	0	0	0	0	—	0	0	0	0
Olives, black	10 extra large	87	0.6	9.5	1.5	0.8	50	355	30	Trace	Trace	—	—
Onions, raw, chopped	1 cup	65	2.6	.2	14.8	0.9	46	17	70	.05	.07	.3	17
Oranges, whole	1, 2⅝ in diam.	64	1.3	.3	16.0	0.5	54	1	260	.13	.05	.5	66
Orange juice	1 cup	112	1.7	.5	25.8	0.5	27	2	500	.22	.07	1.0	124
Pancakes, enriched	1, 4-in diam.	62	1.9	1.9	9.2	0.4	27	115	30	.01	.04	.1	Trace
Parsnips, boiled, diced	1 cup	102	2.3	.8	23.1	0.9	70	12	50	.11	.12	.2	16
Peaches, canned in heavy syrup, sliced	1 cup	200	1.0	.3	51.5	0.8	10	5	1100	.03	.05	1.5	8
Peanuts, roasted in shell	10, jumbo	105	4.7	8.8	3.7	0.4	13	1	—	.06	.02	3.1	0
Peanut butter	1 tbsp	94	4.0	8.1	3.0	0.3	9	97	—	.02	.02	2.4	0
Pears, canned in heavy syrup	1 cup	194	0.5	.5	50.0	0.5	13	3	10	.03	.05	.3	3

Table 9.1 (Continued)

Food	Serving size	Food energy (kcal)	Protein (g)	Fat (g)	Carbo-hydrate (g)	Iron (mg)[a]	Cal-cium (mg)	So-dium (mg)	Vit. A (IU)[b]	Thia-min (mg)	Riboflavin (mg)	Niacin (mg)	Vit. C (mg)
Peas, canned	1 cup	164	8.7	.7	31.1	4.2	50	588	1120	.22	.12	2.2	22
Frozen, cooked	1 cup	109	8.2	.5	18.9	3.0	30	184	960	.43	.14	2.7	21
Peppers, green, raw, chopped	1 cup	33	1.8	.3	7.2	1.1	14	20	630	.12	.12	.8	192
Pickles, dill	1, 4-in	15	0.9	.3	3.0	1.4	35	1928	140	Trace	.03	Trace	8
Sweet	1, 3-in long	51	0.2	.1	12.8	0.4	4	—	30	Trace	.01	Trace	2
Relish	1 tbsp	21	0.1	.1	5.1	0.1	3	107	—	—	—	—	—
Pie, apple, 9-in	1/6 of pie	404	3.5	17.5	60.2	0.5	13	476	50	.03	.03	.6	2
Custard, 9-in	1/6 of pie	331	9.3	16.9	35.6	0.9	146	436	350	.08	.24	.5	0
Lemon me-ringue, 9-in	1/6 of pie	357	5.2	14.3	52.8	0.7	20	395	240	.04	.11	.3	4
Pumpkin, 9-in	1/6 of pie	321	6.1	17.0	37.2	0.8	78	325	3750	.05	.15	.8	Trace
Pineapple, juice pack	1 cup	96	0.7	.2	25.1	0.7	30	2	120	.20	.05	.5	17
Pineapple juice	1 cup	138	1.0	.3	33.8	0.8	38	3	130	.13	.05	.5	23
Pizza, 12-in cheese	1/8 of pizza	147	5.5	4.1	21.9	0.5	86	380	230	.04	.10	.6	4
Plums, canned in heavy syrup	1 cup	214	1.0	.3	55.8	2.3	23	3	3130	.05	.05	1.0	5
Popcorn, plain	1 cup	23	0.8	.3	4.6	0.2	1	Trace	—	.01	.10	0	0
Pork chop, broiled	1 chop (3/lb)	305	19.3	24.7	0	2.7	9	47	0	.75	.22	4.5	—
Pork sausage, cooked	1 link, 1/2 oz	46	2.2	3.9	.2	0.3	1	—	—	—	—	—	—
Potatoes, raw	1 potato (3/lb)	86	2.4	.1	19.2	0.7	8	3	Trace	.11	.05	1.7	23
French fried	10 med. strips	137	2.2	6.6	18.0	0.7	8	3	Trace	.07	.04	1.6	11
Potato chips	10 chips	114	1.1	8.0	10.0	0.4	8	Varia-ble	Trace	.04	.01	1.0	3
Potato salad	1 cup	248	6.8	7.0	40.8	1.5	80	1320	350	.20	.18	2.8	28

Food	Serving size	Food energy (kcal)	Protein (g)	Fat (g)	Carbohydrate (g)	Iron (mg)[a]	Calcium (mg)	Sodium (mg)	Vit. A (IU)[b]	Thiamin (mg)	Riboflavin (mg)	Niacin (mg)	Vit. C (mg)
Pretzels	1 oz	111	2.8	1.3	21.5	0.4	6	476	0	.01	.01	.2	0
Prunes	10 prunes	260	2.1	.6	68.7	4.0	52	8	1630	.09	.17	1.6	3
Prune juice	6 oz	148	0.8	.2	36.5	7.9	27	4	—	.02	.02	.8	4
Pudding, choc., instant with whole milk	1 cup/ from mix	325	7.8	6.5	63.4	1.3	374	322	340	.08	.39	.3	2
Raisins	1 tbsp	26	0.2	Trace	7.0	0.3	6	2	Trace	.01	.01	Trace	Trace
Raspberries, raw	1 cup	70	1.5	.6	16.7	1.1	27	1	160	.04	.11	1.1	31
Rhubarb, raw, diced	1 cup	20	0.7	.1	4.5	1.0	117	2	120	.04	.09	.4	11
Rice, white, cooked, enriched	1 cup	223	4.1	.2	49.6	1.8	21	767	0	.23	.02	2.1	0
Rolls and Buns: Hamburger, hot dog, enriched	1 roll	119	3.3	2.2	21.2	0.8	30	202	Trace	.11	.07	.9	Trace
Hard roll, enriched	1 roll, 1 oz	78	2.5	.8	14.9	0.6	12	156	Trace	.07	.06	.7	Trace
Dinner roll, enriched	1 roll	75	2.1	1.4	13.3	0.5	9	—	Trace	.07	.06	.6	Trace
Salad Dressings: Blue cheese	1 tbsp	76	0.7	7.8	1.1	Trace	12	164	30	Trace	.02	Trace	Trace
French	1 tbsp	66	0.1	6.2	2.8	0.1	2	219	—	—	—	—	—
Italian	1 tbsp	83	Trace	9.0	1.0	Trace	2	314	Trace	Trace	Trace	Trace	—
Thousand Island	1 tbsp	80	0.1	8.0	2.5	0.1	2	112	50	Trace	Trace	Trace	Trace
Salami	1 oz	128	6.7	10.8	.3	1.0	4	—	—	.10	.07	1.5	—
Salmon, pink, canned	1 cup	310	45.1	13.0	0	1.8	431	851	150	.07	.40	17.6	—
Sardines	1 oz	88	5.8	6.9	.2	1.0	100	145	50	.01	.05	1.2	—
Sauerkraut, canned	1 cup	42	2.4	.5	9.4	1.2	85	1755	120	.07	.09	.5	33
Sherbet, orange	1 cup	259	1.7	2.3	59.4	Trace	31	19	120	.02	.06	Trace	4
Shrimp, fried	1 oz	64	5.8	3.1	2.8	0.6	20	53	—	.01	.02	.8	—
Canned	1 cup	148	31.0	1.4	.9	4.0	147	—	80	.01	.04	2.3	—

Table 9.1 (Continued)

Food	Serving size	Food energy (kcal)	Protein (g)	Fat (g)	Carbo-hydrate (g)	Iron (mg)[a]	Cal-cium (mg)	So-dium (mg)	Vit. A (IU)[b]	Thia-min (mg)	Riboflavin (mg)	Niacin (mg)	Vit. C (mg)
Soft drink, cola	12 oz can	144	0	0	36.9	0	0	—	0	0	0	0	0
Soup, canned, un-diluted: Chicken noodle	10½ oz can	158	8.3	4.8	19.7	1.2	21	2432	90	.3	.06	2.1	Trace
Cream of mushroom	10½ oz can	331	5.7	23.8	25.0	0.9	101	2369	180	.03	.30	1.8	Trace
Tomato	10½ oz can	220	4.9	6.4	38.7	1.8	34	2416	2470	.15	.09	2.7	31
Vegetable beef	10½ oz can	198	12.8	5.5	24.1	1.8	31	2605	6710	.09	.12	2.4	—
Soybean curd (tofu)	4 oz	86	9.4	5.0	2.9	2.3	154	8	0	.07	.04	.1	0
Spaghetti, cooked "al dente," en-riched	1 cup	192	6.5	.7	39.1	1.4	14	1	0	.23	.13	1.8	0
Spaghetti w/ meatballs + tom. sauce (canned)	1 cup	258	12.3	10.3	28.5	3.3	53	1220	1000	.15	.18	2.3	5
Spareribs, braised	6.3 oz (from 1 lb)	792	37.4	70.0	0	4.7	16	65	0	.77	.38	6.1	—
Spinach, frozen, leaf	10 oz con-tainer	71	8.5	.9	11.9	7.1	298	151	23000	.28	.45	1.4	99
Squash, summer, cooked	1 cup, cubed	29	1.9	.2	6.5	0.8	53	2	820	.11	.17	1.7	21
Winter, cooked	1 cup, mashed	129	3.7	.8	31.6	1.6	57	2	8610	.10	.27	1.4	27
Strawberries, raw	1 cup, whole	55	1.0	.7	12.5	1.5	31	1	90	.04	.10	.9	88
Sugar, granulated	1 tbsp	46	0	0	12.0	Trace	0	Trace	0	0	0	0	0
Sunflower seed kernels	1 tbsp	50	2.1	4.3	1.8	0.6	11	3	4	.18	.02	.5	0
Sweet potatoes, 5-in long	1 potato	185	2.8	.6	42.6	1.1	52	16	14260	.16	.10	1.0	34
Syrup, table	1 tbsp	59	0	0	15.4	0.8	9	14	—	0	0	0	0
Tangerine	1 large	46	0.8	.2	11.7	0.4	40	2	420	.06	.02	.1	31

Food	Serving size	Food energy (kcal)	Protein (g)	Fat (g)	Carbo-hydrate (g)	Iron (mg)[a]	Cal-cium (mg)	So-dium (mg)	Vit. A (IU)[b]	Thia-min (mg)	Riboflavin (mg)	Niacin (mg)	Vit. C (mg)
Tomatoes, raw	1, 3½ oz	20	1.0	.2	4.3	0.5	12	3	820	.05	.04	.6	21
Canned	1 cup	51	2.4	.5	10.4	1.2	14	313	2170	.12	.07	1.7	41
Tomato juice	1 cup	46	2.2	.2	10.4	2.2	17	486	1940	.12	.07	1.9	39
Tortilla, flour	1, 1 oz	95	2.5	1.8	17.3	1.1	46	—	—	.01	.08	1.0	Trace
Tuna, drained solids, in oil	1 cup	315	46.1	13.1	0	3.0	13	—	130	.08	.19	19.0	—
Turkey, light meat	3 oz	150	28.0	3.3	0	1.0	—	70	—	.04	.12	9.4	—
Dark meat	3 oz	173	25.5	7.1	0	2.0	—	84	—	.03	.20	3.6	—
Turnips, boiled, cubed	1 cup	36	1.2	.3	7.6	0.6	54	53	Trace	.06	.08	.5	34
Turnip greens, boiled	1 cup	29	3.2	.3	5.2	1.6	267	—	9140	.22	.35	.9	100
Veal, braised/ broiled	3 oz	184	23.0	9.4	0	2.7	9	56	—	.06	.21	4.6	—
Waffles, frozen, enriched	1, 1.2 oz	86	2.4	2.1	14.3	0.6	41	219	40	.06	.05	.4	Trace
Watermelon, diced pieces	1 cup	42	0.8	.3	10.2	0.8	11	2	940	.05	.05	.3	11
Wheat flakes, fortified, added sugar, salt	1 cup	106	3.1	.5	24.2	—	12	310	1410	.35	.42	3.5	11
Wheat germ	1 tbsp	23	1.8	.7	3.0	0.5	3	Trace	10	.11	.05	.3	1
Yogurt, plain, whole milk	1 container, 8 oz	140	6.8	7.7	11.1	0.1	251	106	320	.07	.36	.2	2
Plain, from part skim milk	1 container, 8 oz	113	7.7	3.8	11.8	0.1	271	115	150	.09	.41	.2	2

[a]mg, milligrams.
[b]I.U., International Units.
[c]—, data are unreliable.

table gives the values for 1 cup, you will need to divide all nutrient values in half before you record them.

In place of some nutrient values on Table 9.1, you will find a dash instead of a number. This occurs where various samples of a given food were found to have such different amounts of a particular nutrient that it was impossible to select a representative value for the table. For example, there is a dash for the sodium content of salami; most salamis have hundreds of milligrams of sodium per ounce, but there is wide variation in sodium between brands, so no value was given. Of course, when you add a column of figures containing a dash, you must treat the dash as a zero; when that occurs, remember that the sum will be lower than the actual content.

Some common beverages are not listed at all: water, coffee, tea, and diet soda do not appear on the table. Their nutrient content is negligible except for the water they contain, so they can be disregarded here.

If you cannot find an item you consumed on the table, use a value for something similar. For example, if you ate pork and beans (for which there is no listing), use the values for beans and frankfurters; if you ate oatmeal-walnut cookies, you'll come closest by using the values for chocolate chip cookies rather than the values for fig bars or vanilla wafers.

If you cannot find a similar item, list the major ingredients in the food, estimate how much of each was present, and record values for those items. For example, you'll have to put together your own hamburger sandwich by listing the hamburger patty, the roll, and whatever condiments or other ingredients were on it.

Another possible source of nutrient data are the nutrition labels that appear on many packaged foods (Figure 9.2). The top part of the label gives values per serving for kcalories (commonly shown as calories); for grams of protein, carbohydrate, and fat; and for milligrams of sodium. The bottom half of the label lists nutrient content for at least eight nutrients; however, since they are expressed as percentages of recommended intakes, you have to convert them to absolute values to use them in Self-check 9.1.

You can do this by multiplying the percentages by the values shown in Table 9.2, which are referred to as the U.S. Recommended Daily Allowances (U.S. RDA), the standard established for use in nutrition labeling. The U.S. RDA is the standard on which the nutrient percentages on food labels are based; it applies to people from age four through adult, except pregnant and lactating women, whose needs are higher. (Note: The U.S. RDA is not the same thing as the RDA; the U.S. RDA is *derived from* the RDA.)

Table 9.3 gives an example of how to convert label percentages to absolute values; multiply the percentages on the label by the appropriate U.S. RDA values shown in Table 9.2. After you have filled in the values for all the items you consumed, determine the total.

It takes considerable time to analyze your diet by these hand cal-

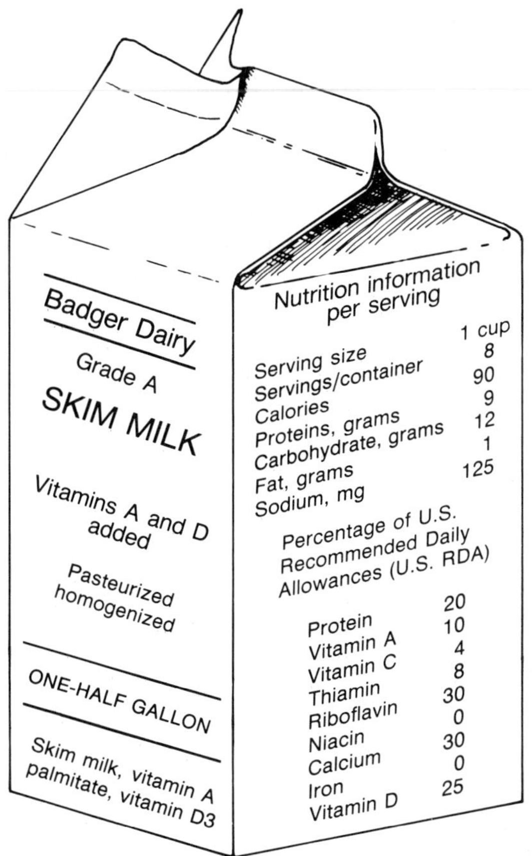

Figure 9.2 A nutrition label. Many packaged foods carry labels that give the nutritional values per serving of the product.

culations, but if you have a computer and some software for diet analysis you can do the job more quickly. (Since the quality of such programs varies substantially, check with a nutritionist knowledgeable in this matter if you plan to purchase diet analysis software.)

Considering Energy Balance

The sum of the first column of figures in Self-check 9.1 tells you how many kcalories you took in on this day. How can you determine whether that amount is right for you?

There is no table that can tell you very accurately how many kcalories you should eat daily. That is because a person's average daily energy intake should be based on his or her average daily energy output, and that varies substantially from one person to another.

Energy output is best estimated on an individual basis, because it is influenced largely by body weight and activity level. Since you have already estimated your energy *output* in Self-check 4.3, you can use that figure here as a basis for judging whether your energy *intake* is appropriate.

If your goal is to keep your body weight constant, your average energy intake and output should match each other, a situation which is referred to as being in *energy balance*. If your goal is to lose weight, your energy intake needs to be less than your output (negative energy balance). To gain weight, kcalorie intake must exceed output (positive energy balance). A pound of fat stores approximately 3500 kcalories; therefore it takes many days of energy imbalance to either gain or lose a pound of fat.

For the present, we will let this brief mention of energy balance suffice, since a later chapter is devoted to a more thorough discussion of this matter.

Table 9.2 The U.S. Recommended Daily Allowances (U.S. RDAs) for 4-year-olds through adults

Nutrient	U.S. RDA
Required on label	
Protein (higher quality)[a]	45 grams
Protein (lower quality)[a]	65 grams
Vitamin A	5000 IU
Vitamin C (ascorbic acid)	60 mg
Thiamin (vitamin B-1)	1.5 mg
Riboflavin (vitamin B-2)	1.7 mg
Niacin	20 mg
Calcium	1.0 grams
Iron	18 mg
Optional on label	
Vitamin D	400 IU
Vitamin E	30 IU
Vitamin B-6	2.0 mg
Folic acid (folacin)	0.4 mg
Vitamin B-12	6 μg
Phosphorus	1.0 grams
Iodine	150 μg
Magnesium	400 mg
Zinc	15 mg
Copper	2 mg
Biotin	0.3 mg
Pantothenic acid	10 mg

[a] Proteins found in food vary in their usefulness to humans. If a particular protein is very good for meeting people's needs, it is called a "high-quality protein," and the 45-gram standard is used. If the protein is of lower quality, the 65-gram standard is used.

Table 9.3   Converting nutrition label percentages to absolute values

Nutrient	% of U.S. RDA	×	U.S. RDA for nutrient	=	Absolute value
Protein	20%	×	45 grams	=	9 grams
Vitamin A	10%	×	5000 IU	=	500 IU
Vitamin C	4%	×	60 mg	=	2.4 mg
Thiamin	8%	×	1.5 mg	=	0.12 mg
Riboflavin	30%	×	1.7 mg	=	0.51 mg
Niacin	0%	×	20 mg	=	0
Calcium	30%	×	1000 mg	=	300 mg
Iron	0%	×	18 mg	=	0
Vitamin D	25%	×	400 IU	=	100 IU

What Were Your Kcalories From?

Not only is the total amount of energy you get from your diet important, but there is also significance in what proportions of energy come from the various nutrients.

Many researchers in nutrition, medicine, and exercise physiology now believe that there are disease prevention and performance benefits associated with consuming certain percentages of energy from protein, fat, and carbohydrate. Many experts believe you can reduce your risk of heart disease and cancer, as well as enhance your ability to perform demanding physical activity day after day, if you distribute your intake of energy nutrients as follows:

- 10 to 15 percent from protein
- 30 percent or less from fat
- 50 to 60 percent from carbohydrate

You can determine what proportion of your energy intake comes from protein, fat, and carbohydrate by following the steps listed in Self-check 9.2. You must multiply the number of grams of protein, fat, and carbohydrate by the kcaloric value per gram for these nutrients (4 kcal/g for protein; 9 kcal/g for fat; and 4 kcal/g for carbohydrate), and then divide each one by the total kcaloric intake. Figure 9.3 gives an example of a filled-out form of Self-check 9.2.

How does your distribution of kcalories match the recommendations given above? Typically, Americans consume more of their energy from fat and less from carbohydrate than is optimal. If you do too, the next chapter will provide some suggestions for food selection that can improve your distribution of kcalories.

Self-check 9.2   Calculating what percentages of energy come from protein, fat, and carbohydrate

	Energy (kcal)	Protein (grams)	Fat (gm)	Carbohydrate (grams)	Alcohol (kcal)
1. Transfer values from Self-check 9.1	A[a]				
2. Multiply by kcal/gram value shown to get energy value		×4	×9	×4	
3. Sum the values in step 2 and record total in space B	B[a] =	+	+		C
4. Divide individual values by total kcalories, which gives decimal fractions					
5. Multiply by 100 to get percentages					

[a]Values in boxes A and B should be within about 25 kcalories of each other. If there is a larger discrepancy, and if there is an alcoholic beverage on the intake record, the extra kcalories are due mainly to the alcohol. To estimate alcohol kcalories, subtract value B from value A and enter the number in box C.

Focusing on Protein Needs

In the section above, we recommended that 10 to 15 percent of kcalories should come from protein; that standard works well for most adults to use for assessing whether their protein intake is appropriate. However, there is a more precise method you can use, which we recommend especially for athletes, pregnant and lactating women, and people who are trying to lose or gain weight. Depending on the situation, the "10 to 15 percent-of-kcalories" guideline may not be appropriate for people who fit these descriptions. Rather, it is more accurate to base recommendations on a certain amount of protein per kilogram of body weight per day.

This method makes use of a person's *best body weight* for calculating recommended dietary protein intake. Your best body weight is the weight at which you know you function best both physically and mentally. It may very well be your present weight or the weight you tend to maintain without effort. If you can't settle on what your best weight is, use the weight suggested for your height from Table 11.1 in Chapter 11. If you are overweight or underweight, it is better to use a "best body weight" figure in the calculation instead of your present weight, because your protein needs to not change significantly with changes

Figure 9.3 An example of using Self-check 9.2 to calculate what percentages of energy come from protein, fat, and carbohydrate. This continues with the example of Lori from Figure 9.1.

	Energy (kcal)	Protein (grams)	Fat (gm)	Carbohydrate (grams)	Alcohol (kcal)
1. Transfer values from Self-check 9.1	A[a] 2274	56	118	252	
2. Multiply by kcal/gram value shown to get energy value		×4 224	×9 1062	×4 1008	
3. Sum the values in step 2 and record total in space B	B[a] 2294 = 224 + 1062 + 1008				C
4. Divide individual values by total kcalories, which gives decimal fractions		.098	.463	.439	
5. Multiply by 100 to get percentages		10%	46%	44%	

[a]Values in boxes A and B should be within about 25 kcalories of each other. If there is a larger discrepancy, and if there is an alcoholic beverage on the intake record, the extra kcalories are due mainly to the alcohol. To estimate alcohol kcalories, subtract value B from value A and enter the number in box C.

in body fat; it is your lean body mass (bone, muscle, skin, organs, etc.) that most influences your protein needs.

Protein needs are higher during growth, since protein is required to construct new tissue. You can see what an influence growth has when you compare the average adult's needs of 0.8 grams of protein/kg of best weight/day (which is only for maintenance of existing tissue) with the needs of the rapidly growing infant for 2.2 grams/kg/day.

Demanding, regular athletic activity is another relevant factor. Athletes may need slightly more protein for repairing the minor injuries that can occur during weight lifting, running, or virtually any demanding physical activity. Also, endurance athletes who exercise continuously for hours at a time (as in running a marathon) may use additional protein for energy, even though under ordinary circumstances our bodies do not use much protein for this purpose. But even when all of these factors are taken into account, the amount of extra protein recommended for athletes is not very large.

This is a surprise to some athletes. Thinking that they need a great deal of extra protein, some athletes eat much more of it than is recommended. They need to know that there may be risks in doing so. Intakes of protein in excess of double the recommendations may pro-

Self-check 9.3   Calculating your recommended daily protein intake

1. Convert best body weight from pounds to kilograms:

$$\text{Body weight in kilograms} = \frac{\text{best body weight (lb)}}{2.2 \text{ lb/kg}} = \frac{\underline{\hspace{2em}} \text{ lb}}{2.2 \text{ lb/kg}} = \underline{\hspace{3em}} \text{ kg}$$

2. Circle the basic standard (and extra need) that applies to you:

Basic standards
Older teen* (nonathlete)	0.85 g/kg body weight
Adult (nonathlete)	0.80 g/kg body weight
Older teen* (athlete)	1.00 g/kg body weight
Adult (athlete)	1.00 g/kg body weight

Extra needs
Pregnant	30 grams more than prepregnant recommendation
Lactating	20 grams more than prepregnant recommendation

3. Calculate the amount of protein recommended for you:
   Recommended daily protein intake
   = (body weight in kg × basic standard) + extra need
   = (_______ kg × _______ grams/kg) + _______ grams
   = _______ grams of protein

*For this purpose, a teen is someone who has grown in height during the past year.

Figure 9.4   A filled-out form of Self-check 9.3 used to calculate recommended daily protein intake. Once again as an example we use Lori, whose one-day intake was shown in Figure 9.1.

1. Convert best body weight from pounds to kilograms:

$$\text{Body weight in kilograms} = \frac{\text{best body weight (lb)}}{2.2 \text{ lb/kg}} = \frac{132 \text{ lb}}{2.2 \text{ lb/kg}} = 60 \text{ kg}$$

2. Circle the basic standard (and extra need) that applies to you:

Basic standards
Older teen* (nonathlete)	0.85 g/kg body weight
Adult (nonathlete)	**(0.80 g/kg body weight)**
Older teen* (athlete)	1.00 g/kg body weight
Adult (athlete)	1.00 g/kg body weight

Extra needs
Pregnant	30 grams more than prepregnant recommendation
Lactating	20 grams more than prepregnant recommendation

3. Calculate the amount of protein recommended for you:
   Recommended daily protein intake
   = (body weight in kg × basic standard) + extra need
   = (60 kg × 0.8 grams/kg) + 0 grams
   = 48 grams of protein

*For this purpose, a teen is someone who has grown in height during the past year.

mote dehydration (an immediate concern) and gradual calcium loss (a long-term concern), and are often accompanied by excessive fat intake (another long-term concern). Furthermore, if a person eats largely high-protein foods and restricts consumption of high-carbohydrate foods, he or she may have less endurance in long distance events; we'll discuss this more thoroughly in the next chapter.

Self-check 9.3 outlines the process and provides a form for calculating your own protein needs. Figure 9.4 offers an example of a filled-out form of Self-check 9.3.

Ideally, your actual protein intake should be close to the level of your recommended protein intake. There are risks of consistently getting either too little protein (less than 70 percent of your recommended intake) or too much (more than double your recommended intake).

If you have calculated your protein needs using both methods—this one and the 10 to 15 percent-of-kcalories method in Self-check 9.2—you may find quite a discrepancy between the recommendations. If you do, consider this latter method as the more accurate of the two; the first one is a rougher estimate.

Are Your Micronutrient Intakes Adequate?

Finally, let's find out how close your intakes of vitamins and minerals are to accepted standards for dietary adequacy.

As you know from the previous chapter, the standard for nutrient intake is the table of Recommended Dietary Allowances (RDAs), shown on Table 9.4. Note that besides the main table, there is an additional table (Table 9.5) called "Estimated safe and adequate daily dietary intakes of selected vitamins and minerals." On that table, values are expressed in ranges, because there is less certainty about what levels of intake are optimal for those nutrients. All of these recommendations are reviewed periodically and revised to reflect new research findings.

Because people's nutrient needs are influenced by gender, age, and reproductive status, there are different intake levels recommended on different lines of the table for various subgroups of people.

Another factor that influences how much of a nutrient you need is individual variability: even within categories, nutrient needs differ somewhat from one individual to another. Considering this, the RDAs are set high enough to include the needs of 98 percent of the normally healthy population. Therefore, if you consume the amounts of nutrients recommended by your RDAs, you are probably taking in more than you actually require for biochemical functions. Note that the RDAs are for healthy people; those who are ill are likely to have higher nutrient needs.

You can compare the amounts of nutrients you consumed with your RDAs by following the instructions in Self-check 9.4. An example is shown in Figure 9.5. This is another function that can also be determined by using special computer software.

Table 9.4   Recommended Dietary Allowances (RDA)

Age (years)	Weight (kg)	Weight (lb)	Height (cm)	Height (in)	Protein (grams)	Fat-soluble vitamins — Vitamin A (μg RE)[a]	Vitamin A (IU)[b]	Vitamin D (μg)	Vitamin D (IU)[b]	Vitamin E (mg α-TE)[c]
Infants										
0.0–0.5	6	13	60	24	kg $\times$ 2.2	420	1400	10	400	3
0.5–1.0	9	20	71	28	kg $\times$ 2.0	400	2000	10	400	4
Children										
1–3	13	29	90	35	23	400	2000	10	400	5
4–6	20	44	112	44	30	500	2500	10	400	6
7–10	28	62	132	52	34	700	3300	10	400	7
Males										
11–14	45	99	157	62	45	1000	5000	10	400	8
15–18	66	145	176	69	56	1000	5000	10	400	10
19–22	70	154	177	70	56	1000	5000	7.5	300	10
23–50	70	154	178	70	56	1000	5000	5	200	10
51+	70	154	178	70	56	1000	5000	5	200	10
Females										
11–14	46	101	157	62	46	800	4000	10	400	8
15–18	55	120	163	64	46	800	4000	10	400	8
19–22	55	120	163	64	44	800	4000	7.5	300	8
23–50	55	120	163	64	44	800	4000	5	200	8
51+	55	120	163	64	44	800	4000	5	200	8
Pregnant					+30	+200	+1000	+5	+200	+2
Lactating					+20	+400	+2000	+5	+200	+3

[a]Retinol equivalents.
[b]International units. On the official 1980 RDA table, recommended intakes of vitamins A and D are not expressed in IUs, as they had been in prior editions. They are added here for comparison.
[c]Alpha tocopherol.
[d]Niacin equivalents.
[e]The increased requirement during pregnancy cannot be met by the iron content of habitual American diets nor by the existing iron stores of many women; therefore the use of 30–60 mg of supplemental iron is recommended. Iron needs during lactation are not substantially different from those of nonpregnant women, but continued supplementation of the mother for 2–3 months after delivery is advisable in order to replenish stores depleted by pregnancy.

After you have done the calculation, you need to interpret your findings: that is, how important is it to take in 100 percent of the RDA each day?

As explained above, most healthy people's actual nutrient needs are less than the levels recommended by the RDA; you might very well meet your biochemical need for a particular nutrient with an intake of less than 100 percent of the RDA. Therefore, many experts in nutritional assessment judge a diet to be generally adequate if it contains *at least 70 percent of the RDA for all nutrients.*

Table 9.4 Continued

Age (years)	Water-soluble vitamins							Minerals					
	Vit. C (mg)	Thiamin (mg)	Riboflavin (mg)	Niacin (mg NE)[d]	Vit. B-6 (mg)	Folacin (µg)	Vit. B-12 (µg)	Calcium (mg)	Phosphorus (mg)	Magnesium (mg)	Iron (mg)	Zinc (mg)	Iodine (µg)
Infants													
0.0–0.5	35	0.3	0.4	6	0.3	30	0.5	360	240	50	10	3	40
0.5–1.0	35	0.5	0.6	8	0.6	45	1.5	540	360	70	15	5	50
Children													
1–3	45	0.7	0.8	9	0.9	100	2.0	800	800	150	15	10	70
4–6	45	0.9	1.0	11	1.3	200	2.5	800	800	200	10	10	90
7–10	45	1.2	1.4	16	1.6	300	3.0	800	800	250	10	10	120
Males													
11–14	50	1.4	1.6	18	1.8	400	3.0	1200	1200	350	18	15	150
15–18	60	1.4	1.7	18	2.0	400	3.0	1200	1200	400	18	15	150
19–22	60	1.5	1.7	19	2.2	400	3.0	800	800	350	10	15	150
23–50	60	1.4	1.6	18	2.2	400	3.0	800	800	350	10	15	150
51+	60	1.2	1.4	16	2.2	400	3.0	800	800	350	10	15	150
Females													
11–14	50	1.1	1.3	15	1.8	400	3.0	1200	1200	300	18	15	150
15–18	60	1.1	1.3	14	2.0	400	3.0	1200	1200	300	18	15	150
19–22	60	1.1	1.3	14	2.0	400	3.0	800	800	300	18	15	150
23–50	60	1.0	1.2	13	2.0	400	3.0	800	800	300	18	15	150
51+	60	1.0	1.2	13	2.0	400	3.0	800	800	300	10	15	150
Pregnant	+20	+0.4	+0.3	+2	+0.6	+400	+1.0	+400	+400	+150	e	+5	+25
Lactating	+40	+0.5	+0.5	+5	+0.5	+100	+1.0	+400	+400	+150	e	+10	+50

What are the guidelines for the *upper* limits? It's tempting to say that a certain multiple of the RDA—such as 10 times the RDA—is the point at which nutrients become toxic. That would be an easy value to remember and apply, but it would not be accurate. For most nutrients, we don't yet know at what level harm is likely. For those we do know about, we see considerable variation in toxicity levels. For one nutrient—for example, vitamin D—an intake of 300 percent (three times the RDA) could lead to difficulties if continued for an extended time; for another—for example, vitamin C—negative effects are not likely to occur unless much larger excesses are consumed. This disparity makes it difficult to set a limit factor that can be applied to all nutrients. The key point is that *more is not better; there is no known advantage for a healthy person to consume more than 100 percent of the RDA.* Even a nutrient as heavily marketed as vitamin C has a point at which it is toxic.

Table 9.5   Estimated safe and adequate daily dietary intakes of selected vitamins and minerals[a]

	Age (years)	Vitamins		
		Vitamin K (μg)	Biotin (μg)	Pantothenic acid (mg)
Infants	0–0.5	12	35	2
	0.5–1	10–20	50	3
Children and	1–3	15–30	65	3
adolescents	4–6	20–40	85	3–4
	7–10	30–60	120	4–5
	11+	50–100	100–200	4–7
Adults		70–140	100–200	4–7

	Age (years)	Trace elements[b]					
		Copper (mg)	Manganese (mg)	Fluoride (mg)	Chromium (mg)	Selenium (mg)	Molybdenum (mg)
Infants	0–0.5	0.5–0.7	0.5–0.7	0.1–0.5	0.01–0.04	0.01–0.04	0.03–0.06
	0.5–1	0.7–1.0	0.7–1.0	0.2–1.0	0.02–0.06	0.02–0.06	0.04–0.08
Children and	1–3	1.0–1.5	1.0–1.5	0.5–1.5	0.02–0.08	0.02–0.08	0.05–0.1
adolescents	4–6	1.5–2.0	1.5–2.0	1.0–2.5	0.03–0.12	0.03–0.12	0.06–0.15
	7–10	2.0–2.5	2.0–3.0	1.5–2.5	0.05–0.2	0.05–0.2	0.10–0.3
	11+	2.0–3.0	2.5–5.0	1.5–2.5	0.05–0.2	0.05–0.2	0.15–0.5
Adults		2.0–3.0	2.5–5.0	1.5–4.0	0.05–0.2	0.05–0.2	0.15–0.5

	Age (years)	Electrolytes		
		Sodium (mg)	Potassium (mg)	Chloride (mg)
Infants	0–0.5	115–350	350–925	275–700
	0.5–1	250–750	425–1275	400–1200
Children and	1–3	325–975	550–1650	500–1500
adolescents	4–6	450–1350	775–2325	700–2100
	7–10	600–1800	1000–3000	925–2775
	11+	900–2700	1525–4575	1400–4200
Adults		1100–3300	1875–5625	1700–5100

[a]Because there is less information available on which to base allowances, these figures are not given in the main table of the RDA and are provided here in the form of ranges of recommended intakes.
[b]Since the toxic levels for many trace elements may be only several times usual intakes, the upper levels for the trace elements given in this table should not be habitually exceeded.

Now that you have evaluated your diet in various ways, you should have some sense of whether your eating style promotes good health. But remember not to put too much weight on your analysis of just one day: the more days you analyze, the more accurate your results will be.

If your current diet does not rate very favorably, the next chapter should be of particular interest to you: it offers a guide for selecting foods that can help you progress toward a healthier eating style.

Self-check 9.4   Comparing your actual vitamin and mineral intakes with your Recommended Dietary Allowances or RDAs

	Iron (mg)	Calcium (mg)	Sodium (mg)	Vitamin A (IU)	Thiamin (vitamin B-1) (mg)	Riboflavin (vitamin B-2) (mg)	Niacin (mg)	Vitamin C (ascorbic acid) (mg)
1. Enter totals from Self-check 9.1								
2. Enter RDAs from Table 9.3								
3. Divide totals by RDAs								
4. Multiply by 100 to get percentage								

Figure 9.5   An example of how to compare your vitamin and mineral intakes with your Recommended Dietary Allowances, or RDAs (a completed Self-check 9.4). Again we use the example of Lori, who was introduced in Figure 9.1.

	Iron (mg)	Calcium (mg)	Sodium (mg)	Vitamin A (IU)	Thiamin (vitamin B-1) (mg)	Riboflavin (vitamin B-2) (mg)	Niacin (mg)	Vitamin C (ascorbic acid) (mg)
1. Enter totals from Self-check 9.1	9.9	663	4395	4455	1.10	2.04	11.5	20
2. Enter RDAs from Table 9.3	18.0	800	1100–3300	4000	1.1	1.3	14	60
3. Divide totals by RDAs	.55	.829	1.331	1.113	1.00	1.569	.821	.333
4. Multiply by 100 to get percentage	55%	83%	133%	111%	100%	157%	82%	33%

Food for Health, Performance, and Pleasure 10

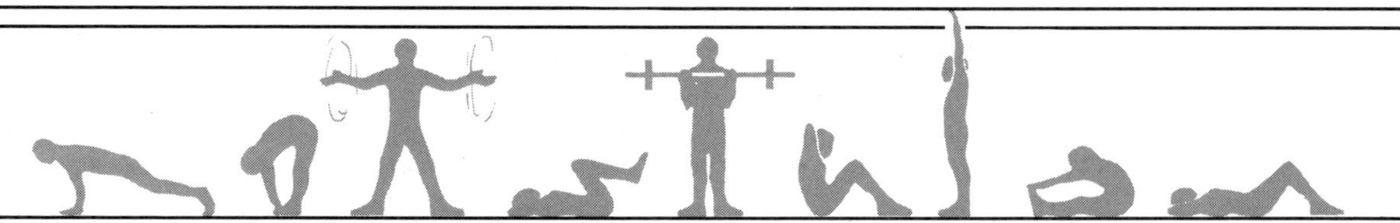

Outline

When you rated your diet in the last chapter, how did it fare? Did you find some characteristics that were less than ideal?

If your diet was the meat-and-potatoes type like Mike's (you met him at the beginning of Chapter 9), it was probably higher in fat and lower in vitamins A and C than is recommended. If you identified with weight-conscious Beth, your kcalorie, carbohydrate, and various other nutrient intakes were probably very low on dieting days, but you may have more than made up for the intended energy shortfall on other days. Are you a lacto-ovo-vegetarian like Aaron? Your diet may have been low in iron. Julie may have come out the best overall on her rating (especially if she averaged several days), since she practices one

"

of the most important guidelines for being well nourished—getting a lot of variety in her diet.

Few people have food habits that are absolutely ideal; almost everybody finds some way in which their nutrition could be improved. For those who see the need for some changes, this chapter can help out.

In the nutrition basics and assessment chapters, we focused largely on nutrients and what they do for you. Here we will concentrate more on the foods that provide the nutrients, since that focus can help guide your choices in a restaurant, a grocery store, or a cafeteria line—places where your nutrition is directly affected.

The recommendations you will find here are based on getting enough of the essential nutrients, as well as limiting the intake of certain dietary components that are risk factors for disease.

In addition, we will deal with the question of who needs nutritional supplements, and offer general guidelines for their use. We will also describe how athletes can improve performance through optimal nutrition.

If all this sounds very clinical, rest assured that we haven't forgotten that eating is one of life's pleasures. You don't need to sacrifice enjoyment as you make your habits healthier. But you do have to go slowly enough in making changes (as described in Chapter 2) so you can enjoy your new, gradually evolving eating style.

Let's begin by looking at a simple system that is a useful guide for what to eat from day to day.

Using the Basic Food Guide

When you used the food composition table, you probably noticed that certain foods have nutritional similarities. For example, plain yogurt resembles milk; meats are quite similar to one another in nutrient content; and fruits and vegetables share many characteristics with one another.

Based on such similar nutritional attributes, we can assign many foods to four major groups—dairy products, grain products, meats and meat alternates, and fruits and vegetables. Table 10.1 identifies a few of the nutrients furnished in significant amounts by the foods in these groups. It is possible to achieve adequate nutrient intakes by consuming enough foods from each of these groups daily.

Those factors are the basis of eating guides, such as the Basic Four Food Guide, which was published by the U.S. Department of Agriculture in 1956 and has been widely used ever since. Here we offer an adaptation of the Basic Four which we simply call the *Basic Food Guide*. The advantage this guide offers over the Basic Four Food Guide is that in addition to recommendations about how many servings of food to eat from each group, the Basic Food Guide provides information regarding how much fat, sodium, and added sugar are present in var-

Table 10.1   The four basic food groups and some nutrients they provide

Food groups	Examples	A few of the nutrients present in significant amounts
Fruits and vegetables	Apples, bananas, cherries, dates, etc.; asparagus, broccoli, cauliflower, green beans, squash, etc.	Vitamins A and/or C in some items Carbohydrate Water Some B vitamins
Grain products	Breads, cereals, pasta, rice	Carbohydrate Some B vitamins
Milk products	Milk, yogurt, cheese, ice cream	Protein Calcium and phosphorus Some B vitamins
Meats and alternates	Beef, chicken, fish, eggs, nuts, navy beans	Protein Iron and zinc Some B vitamins

ious foods within each group—information which the Basic Four does not provide.

The six food groups of the Basic Food Guide are shown in Figures 10.1 through 10.6.

The four basic food groups

Shown near the top of Figures 10.1 through 10.4 are the minimal daily intake recommendations for adults for the first four basic food groups. You should consume *at least* as much each day as these guidelines suggest; most people will consume more, since the minimum recommendations by themselves are not likely to provide enough food to meet most people's energy needs for a day. When you need more food to satisfy hunger than the minimums suggest, it's better to eat more of these basic foods than to eat a lot of other things that aren't very nourishing. We'll talk more about these less-nourishing foods (we call them "limited extras") shortly.

On each of these four figures you will notice that there are serving sizes given for some representative foods within each group. For foods that are not shown but seem very similar to others there, you can assume the serving size will be the same.

Of course, people sometimes eat more or less of these foods at one time than our serving sizes suggest, and that's fine. These reference serving sizes are primarily a tool for helping people determine their appropriate total intake for the day. Therefore, it's fine to drink just a half cup of milk at a time even though the Basic Food Guide serving

Figure 10.1

Fruits and Vegetables

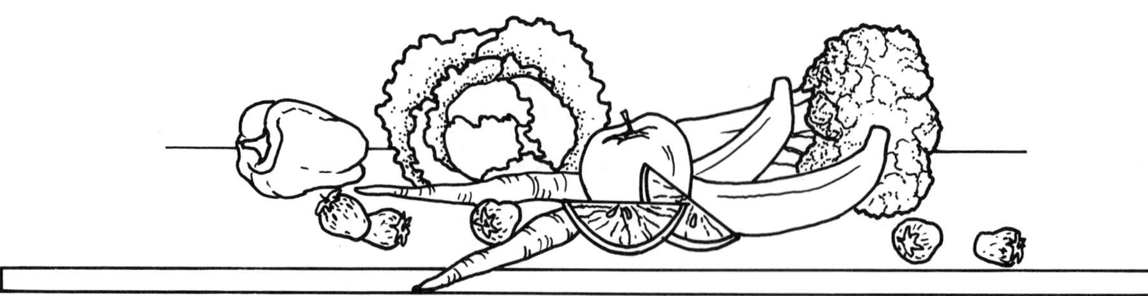

You need at least four servings daily, including:

One good source of vitamin A—*apricots, broccoli, cantaloupe, carrots, pumpkin, winter squash, sweet potatoes, spinach and other dark, leafy greens.*

One good source of vitamin C—*broccoli, cabbage, cantaloupe, cauliflower, grapefruit, green pepper, lemons, limes, oranges, strawberries, tangerines.*

Each of these is a serving:
½ cup fresh, frozen, or canned solid product
1 medium-sized piece of fruit (e.g., apple, orange, banana)
½ cup fresh, frozen, or canned juice
1 cup raw vegetables
¼ cup dried fruits or vegetables

How much fat, sodium, and added sugar are likely to be found in fruit and vegetable products?

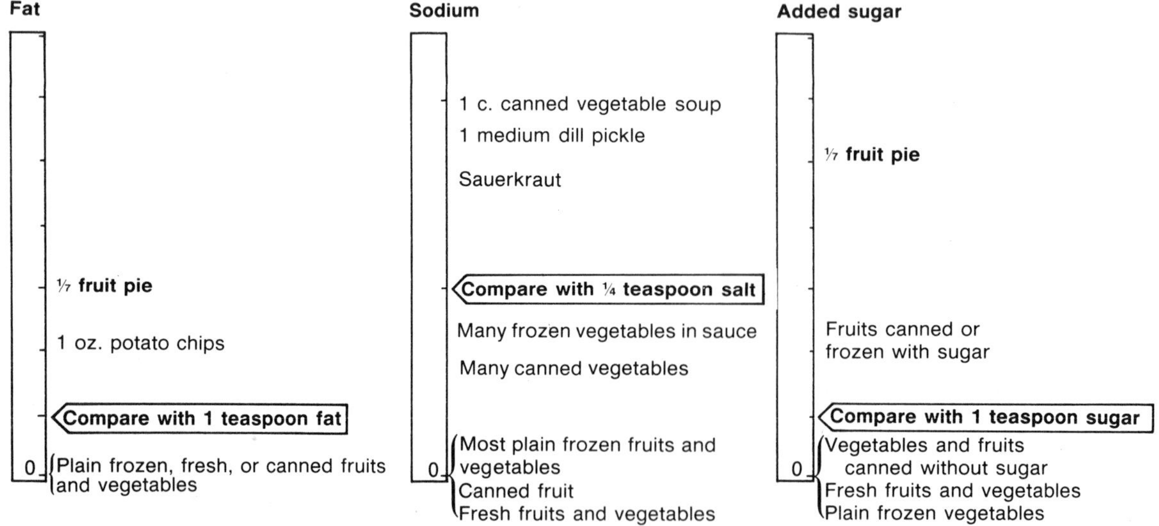

Figure 10.2

Grain products

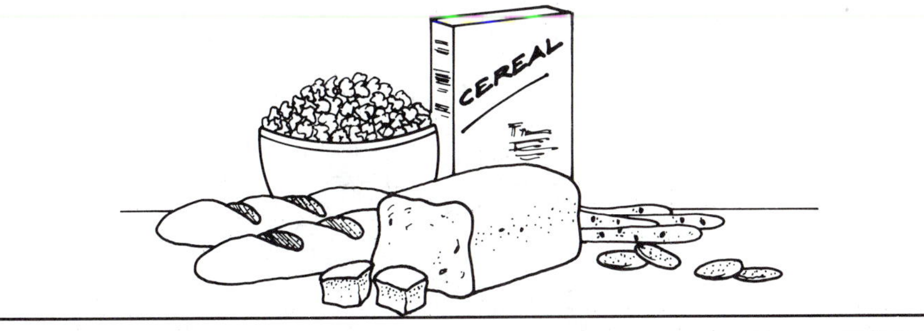

You need at least four servings daily, including:

two whole-grain products; *other servings should be enriched or fortified.*

Each of these is a serving:

1 slice of bread or medium dinner roll
½ hamburger or hot-dog bun
½ English muffin
2½ tablespoons flour
1 oz. dry cereal
½ cup cooked cereal

3 cups popped popcorn
1 tortilla, pancake, or waffle
½ cup cooked pasta, rice, or
    other grain
6 Saltines, snack crackers, or pretzels
3 graham crackers or unfrosted cookies

How much fat, sodium, and added sugar are likely to be found in grain products?

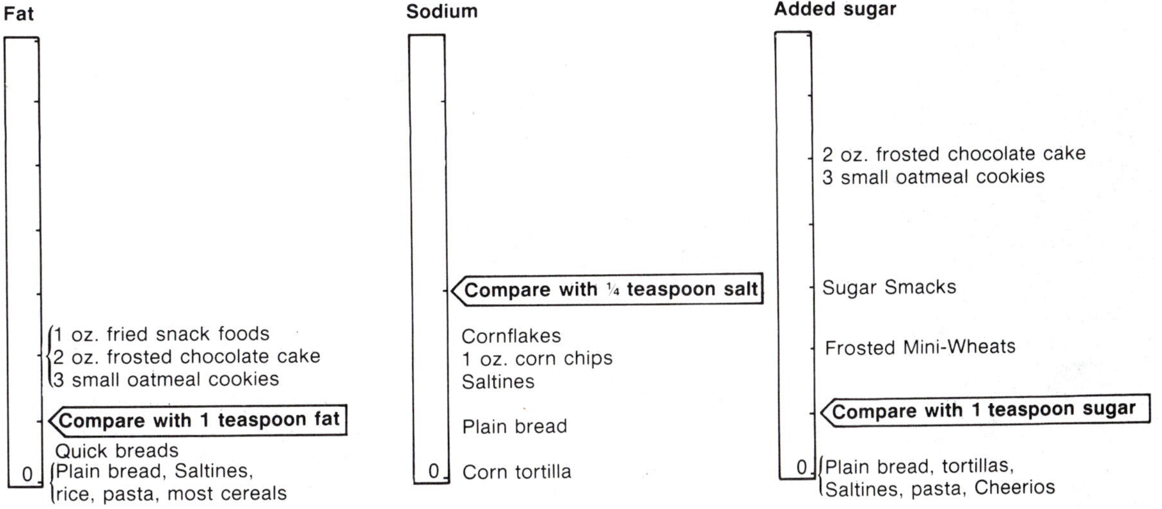

Figure 10.3

Milk and Milk Products

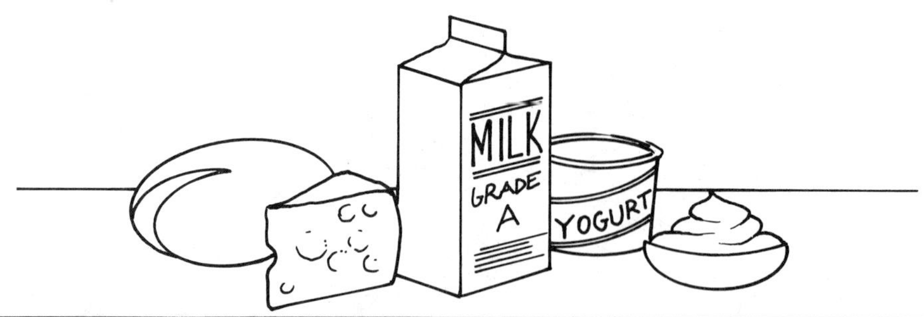

Adults need at least two servings daily. Teens need four servings daily; children from 9 to 12 years old need three servings; children under 9 years old need two to three servings.

Each of these is a serving:
1 cup milk or yogurt
1⅓ oz. hard cheese
2 oz. processed cheese food
2 cups cottage cheese
1 cup sauce or pudding made with milk
1½ cups ice cream or ice milk

How much fat, sodium, and added sugar are likely to be found in milk and milk products?

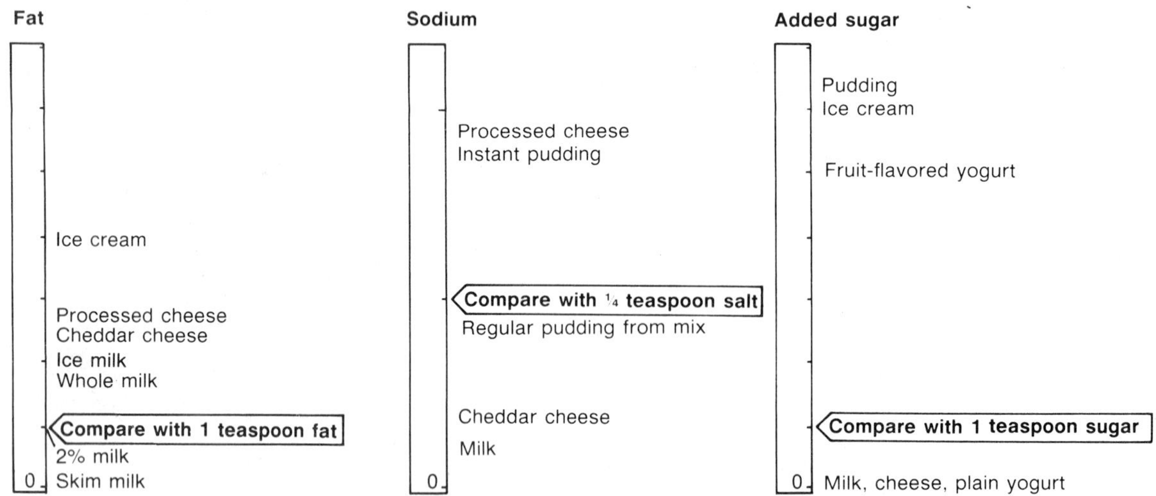

Figure 10.4

Meats and Alternates

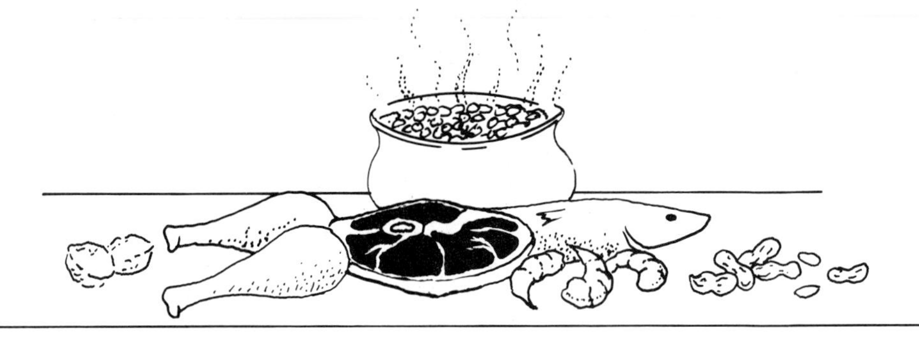

You need at least two servings daily, including:

plant sources several times a week.

Each of these is a serving:
2 to 3 oz. lean, boneless cooked meat, fish, or poultry
   (a piece the size of the palm of your hand, and ⅜ inch thick)

The following can substitute for 2 oz. of meat:
2 eggs
1 cup cooked legumes (e.g., black, garbanzo, kidney, lima,
   navy, pinto, or soy beans; lentils; split peas)
6 oz. tofu
2 oz. (approximately ½ cup) nuts or seeds
2 oz. (approximately ¼ cup) nut or seed butter

How much fat, sodium, and added sugar are likely to be found in meat and alternates?

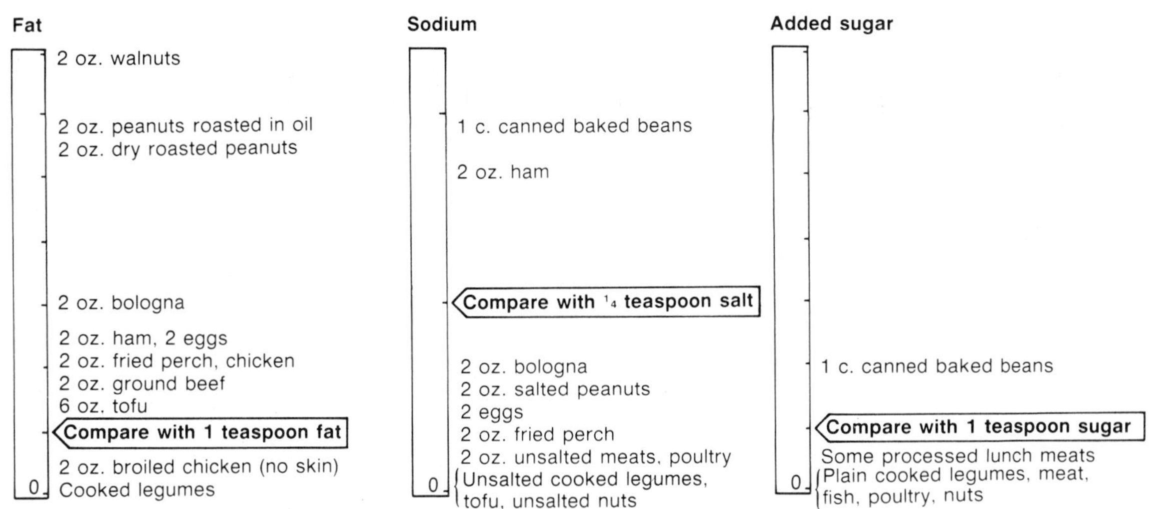

size is 1 cup; just realize that the half cup represents one-fourth of the day's total of two servings recommended for an adult.

At the bottom of each food group figure are vertical lines (or rulers) labeled "fat," "sodium," and "added sugar." Here you can see how much of these substances are in some representative foods in each group. The bottom of each ruler represents zero, with values increasing as you ascend. Some foods from the group are placed along each ruler, showing the relative content of fat, sodium, and added sugar. For the sake of comparison, a specific amount of pure fat, salt, and sugar are also indicated along the rulers. If you want to reduce the amounts of these substances in your diet, you can do so by eating more foods from nearer the bottom of the rulers, and fewer foods from higher up.

Combination foods

Figure 10.5 shows how to deal with combination foods such as casseroles or soups when you use this system. First you should mentally separate the foods into their components; then identify which groups the ingredients belong to; and finally estimate what part of a serving each represents. Some common examples are shown. Using these as guidelines, you can estimate other combination foods in your diet for yourself.

Limited extras

Figure 10.6 deals with the limited extras, popularly referred to as "junk food." These are consumables that generally have very low micronutrient content but a considerable number of kcalories due to high levels of fat and/or added sugar. Some are also high in sodium.

In nutritional terms, a few servings of limited extras per day are tolerable, but you should not eat large amounts of these foods. If you do, you are likely to get excessive amounts of fat, sodium, and added sugar; furthermore, you may not get enough of the essential nutrients. If you want more to eat, rely primarily on additional foods from the four basic groups.

These are the limited extras:

- Fatty foods: butter, cream, sour cream, cream cheese, bacon, lard and other solid shortenings, mayonnaise, cooking oil, oil-based salad dressings, margarine
- Sugary foods: white, brown, or raw sugar; honey; syrup; molasses; jam or jelly; sugar-sweetened soft drinks; gelatin desserts; other sweet desserts
- Refined, unenriched, or unfortified grain products: breads, crackers, cereals, cookies, cakes, or fried snack foods that are not made from whole, enriched, or fortified grains
- Alcoholic beverages (avoid during pregnancy): beer, wine, hard liquor, liqueur

Figure 10.5

Combination Foods

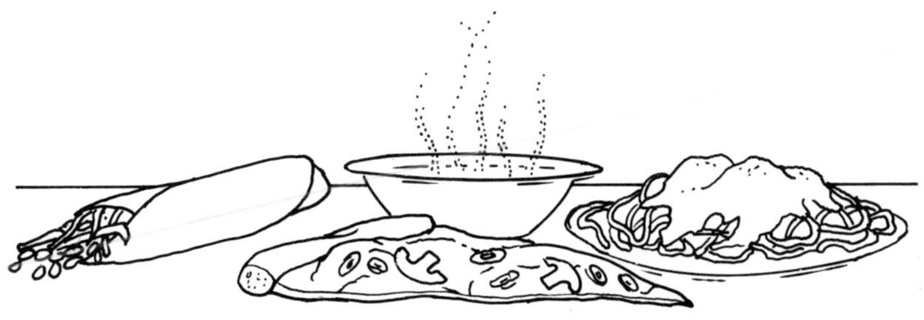

The basic food guide can be used to evaluate a combination food: Mentally separate the food into its ingredients and estimate the amounts of the basic foods present. The following examples show how to analyze some combination foods and can be used as guidelines for analyzing other foods:

¼ of 12-inch cheese pizza
2 oz. cheese = 1½ servings milk
pizza dough = 3 servings grain
¼ c. vegetables = ½ serving vegetable

1 cup chicken chow mein
2 oz. meat = 1 serving meat
½ c. vegetables = 1 serving vegetable

1 cup spaghetti with meatballs
2 oz. meat = 1 serving meat
¾ c. spaghetti = 1½ servings grain
¼ c. tomato sauce = ½ serving vegetable

One 6-ounce bean burrito
½ c. beans = ½ serving meat alternate
1 tortilla = 1 serving grain

1 cup macaroni and cheese
1 oz. cheese = ¾ serving milk
1 c. macaroni = 2 servings grain
2 oz. milk = ¼ serving milk

1 cup canned beef noodle soup
½ oz. meat = ¼ serving meat
¼ c. noodles = ½ serving grain

How much fat, sodium, and added sugar are likely to be found in combination foods?

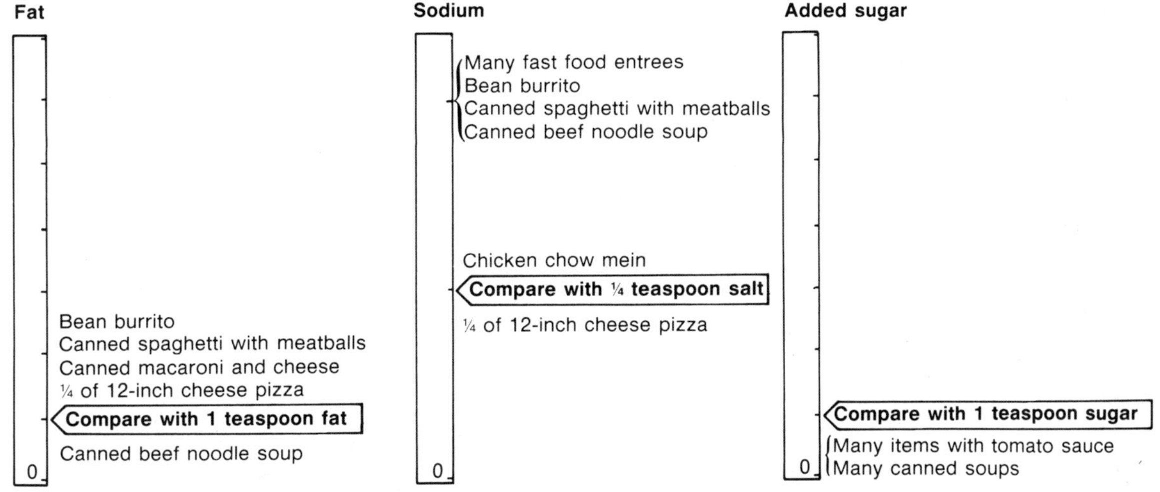

Figure 10.6

Limited Extras

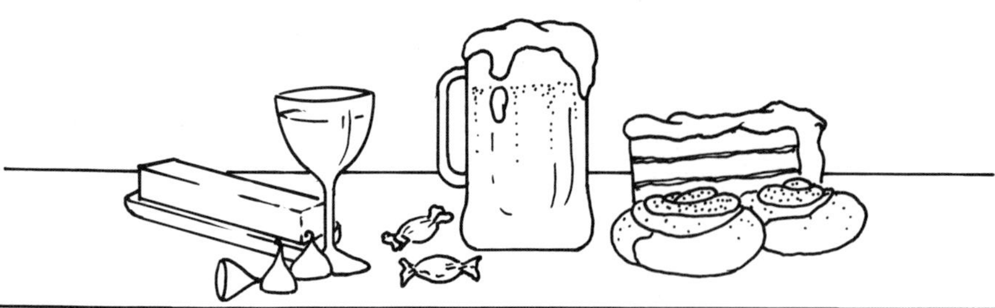

These foods are not needed for good nutrition.

They are not included in the four food groups because they do not contain the essential nutrients in significant amounts. This doesn't mean that they should never be eaten, but they should be used only as limited extras, rather than as mainstays of the diet.

Many of these limited extras have kcalories that add up quickly (fatty and sugary foods, alcoholic beverages, and unenriched baked goods). If you are overweight, you can cut kcalories by eating fewer of these foods. If you are at a good weight for your height and build, it is reasonable to eat some of these foods, provided that you have included all the recommended foods as the basis of your daily diet.

Some items shown along the rulers below have both low kcalories and low nutrient levels. Tea, coffee, broth, low-kcalorie soft drinks, and diet gelatin desserts are in this category. Although they are low in most essential nutrients, they do contribute water.

What are you getting out of your limited extras?

Fatty foods

- 1 oz. Italian salad dressing
- 1⅓ oz. cream cheese
- 1 oz. French dressing
- 2 slices bacon, 1 oz. chocolate
- 1 t. oil, 2 T. sour cream
- **Compare with 1 teaspoon fat**
- 1 t. butter, margarine, lard, shortening, mayonnaise

Alcoholic beverages

- **Compare with 1 oz. alcohol**
- 6 oz. wine
- 1½ oz. liquor
- 12 oz. beer

Salty foods

- 1 T. soy sauce
- 1 c. broth
- ½ t. meat tenderizer
- 1 T. teriyaki sauce
- **Compare with ¼ teaspoon salt**
- 1 oz. French dressing
- 1 oz. Italian dressing
- 4 green olives
- 2 slices bacon
- 1 T. catsup

Sugary foods

- 12 oz. cola beverages
- ½ c. sherbet
- ½ c. gelatin dessert
- 1 T. honey
- 1 T. syrup, ½ oz. hard candy
- 1 T. molasses
- 1 oz. chocolate candy
- 1 t. jam, jelly
- **Compare with 1 teaspoon sugar**

Refined, unenriched baked goods

- 2 oz. pound cake
- 1 Danish pastry
- 3 oz. cheesecake
- 2 oz. brownie with icing
- 1 glazed donut
- 2 oz. banana bread
- 1 oz. baking powder biscuit
- **100 kcalories**
- 1½ oz. Boston brown bread
- 1 slice wheat or rye bread

- Foods that are low in both kcalories and essential nutrients: coffee, tea, broth, some artificially sweetened products such as diet soft drinks and diet gelatin desserts, condiments

Using the food group information

Tables 10.2 and 10.3 summarize information about how many servings of foods from the four basic groups are needed by healthy people each day. They give recommendations for people of various ages, conditions, and lifestyles, such as pregnant and lactating women, athletes, vegetarians, and people on a tight budget.

Once you know the Basic Food Guide groups, serving sizes, and recommended minimum numbers of servings that apply to you, you can use this information to help yourself make more nutritious food selections. For example, if you customarily eat more than ten servings of grain products daily but only two or three servings of fruits and vegetables, the Basic Food Guide recommendations suggest that you might substitute a piece of fresh fruit as a snack instead of your usual package of cheese crackers. Or when you arrive at the cafeteria for supper, you can mentally tally up what you have eaten so far that day, and quickly use the Basic Food Guide to decide what items will fulfill your remaining needs for the day.

Table 10.2   Basic food guide recommendations for various ages and reproductive statuses

	Include at least this many servings daily				
	Child ½–9 years	Child 9–12 years	Teen[a]	Adult[a]	Pregnant or lactating
Fruits and vegetables [b]					
Vitamin A rich	1	1	1	1	1
Vitamin C rich	1	1	1	1	2
Others	2	2	2	2	2
Total	4	4	4	4	5
Grain products (preferably whole grain; otherwise enriched or fortified)	4[c]	4	4	4	4 or more for adequate weight gain
Milk and milk products	2–3	3	4	2	4[e]
Meats and alternates	2[d]	2	2	2	3

[a]A *teen* is defined as a person who has added height in the past year and is at least 12 years old; an *adult* has not added height in that time.
[b]For preschool children, serving size is 1 tablespoon per year of age.
[c]Give smaller servings, depending on age.
[d]For preschool children, serving size is half of the standard serving.
[e]For pregnant teenagers, increase to 5 servings.

Table 10.3   Basic food guide recommendations for certain lifestyles

| | Include at least this many servings daily | | | |
| | Athletes | Adult vegetarians | | Adults with limited budget |
	Teen Adult	Who use milk	Who use only plant foods	
Fruits and vegetables	Fruits/vegetables: 1 vitamin A 1 vitamin C Others to make group total of 4	Fruits:1–4, including 1 raw vitamin C Vegetables: 3, including 1 or more dark leafy green	Fruits:1–4, including 1 raw vitamin C Vegetables: 4, including 2 or more dark leafy green	Fruits/vegetables: 1 vitamin A 1 vitamin C Others to make group total of 4
Grain products	4–12 or more as needed for energy	Whole grain yeast bread: 3 slices Other grains: 2	Whole grain yeast bread: 4 slices Other grains: 3–5	9–12
Milk and milk products	4 (teen) 2 (adult)	2	0	1½
Meats and alternates	2	Legumes: 1 serving Nuts or seeds: ½ serving	Nuts or seeds: 1 serving { Fortified soybean milk: 2 cups Legumes: ⅓ cup *or* { Legumes: 1¼ cup Good sources of vitamin B-12[a] and calcium[b]	2

[a]Good sources of vitamin B-12 are: fortified soy milk, fortified nutritional yeast, vitamin supplement (Robertson, 1976).
[b]Good sources of calcium are: fortified soy milk, some leafy greens, sunflower seeds, unhulled sesame seeds, blackstrap molasses (Robertson, 1976).

Using the rulers

Here are examples of how to use the rulers to monitor and modify your intakes of fat, sodium, and added sugar.

Let's say that when you assessed what proportions of your energy intake came from protein, fat, and carbohydrate (as described in Chapter 9), you learned that you consumed too much fat.

One approach to lowering your fat consumption would be to look at the fat rulers in Figures 10.1 through 10.6 to see what levels of fat are in the foods you consumed. Look at the limited extras first: are you eating many that are high in fat? If so, it would make good sense to

Table 10.4   Recommended daily limits for fat, added sugar, and sodium intake based on the typical number of kcalories consumed per day

	For person with total daily intake of				
	1500 kcal	2000 kcal	2500 kcal	3000 kcal	4000 kcal
Fat[a]	10 teaspoons	13 teaspoons	17 teaspoons	20 teaspoons	27 teaspoons
Added sugar [b]	9 teaspoons	13 teaspoons	16 teaspoons	19 teaspoons	25 teaspoons
Sodium	For all levels, the recommended limit is equal to the amount in ½–1½ teaspoons of salt[c]				

[a]Based on 30% of total kilocalorie consumption.
[b]Based on 10% of total kilocalorie consumption.
[c]Equivalent to safe and adequate range of 1100–3300 mg of sodium.

begin by gradually reducing your intake of those items. Then look at your consumption of foods in the basic food groups: are you eating many items that are high on the fat rulers, while bypassing those lower down? If so, some substitutions would be in order.

Table 10.4 will help you to arrive at reasonable maximum limits for your daily consumption of fat, sugar, and salt, depending on the total number of kcalories you typically consume. Since each mark on the fat and sugar rulers represents one teaspoon, and each mark on the sodium ruler stands for the sodium in 1/4 teaspoon of salt, you can quickly add up how much of these substances you are likely to get in your diet. If you take in too much of any of them, you can use the rulers to suggest substitutions that would bring you closer to your goals.

Food Handling for Nutriton

Another factor that affects the nutritional benefit you get from food is the type and amount of processing it has been subjected to.

Of all the classes of nutrients, vitamins are the most vulnerable. Certain vitamins can be destroyed by oxygen, light, heat, length of storage, or the pH (the acidity or alkalinity) of the food it is part of. As mentioned in Chapter 8, commercial processors make every effort to minimize these losses, but they are unavoidable to a certain degree.

The very best nutrient contents are found in foods that have just been harvested. The next-highest levels are found in frozen and in rapidly dehydrated foods (commercial processes other than sun-drying), followed by canned and by slowly dehydrated foods (sun-drying and home-drying processes). However, even with the more nutrient-destructive processes, approximately half of the original vitamin level is retained.

Another consideration is how you store and handle food after you get it home. Because the way we handle food at home is less carefully controlled than it is commercially, nutrient losses are probably larger at home. It is important to store food properly—especially fresh food—

Table 10.5 Maintaining higher nutrient levels

Foods	When purchasing	During storage	During preparation
All kinds	Very fresh products have highest levels, followed by frozen, rapidly dehydrated, canned, and slowly dehydrated foods	Whether fresh or preserved, vitamin content is higher if food is used sooner and stored cooler Frozen foods retain vitamins best at 0°F and below	If cutting up, delay until necessary If cooking, heat only long enough to be *done* Use minimal amount of water for cooking
Fruits and vegetables		Wrap tightly to exclude air if item doesn't have protective peeling Keep whole Keep cold	Use edible parts known to have high nutrient level If cooking, cook without water or for shortest possible time in least possible water
Grain products	Whole grains have higher nutrient levels than refined products Enriched products are better than refined Fortified cereals have variable nutrient contents		Cook cereals and rice in just enough water to be absorbed
Dairy products	Plastic and cardboard containers conserve nutrients better than clear glass ones do	Keep cold Keep covered Keep away from strong light	
Meats	Fresh meats have a higher vitamin content than smoked ones Expense does not correspond to nutrient value	Keep cold	Use meat drippings (not the melted fat)

to keep as much of the nutrient value as possible. The best general guidelines are to wrap food tightly and to keep it in a dark, cold place.

How you prepare food is also important. The more you peel, cut, and cook food, the greater the vitamin losses will be. Minimizing food handling, cutting things up just before you will use them, and cooking as briefly as possible with little or no water helps preserve vitamin values.

Table 10.5 summarizes recommended practices for purchasing, storing, and preparing foods.

Do You Need Nutritional Supplements?

According to national surveys, almost half the people in the United States take vitamin and/or mineral supplements. Is this really necessary?